Keto Diet Complete Guide:
3 Books in 1:

Your Ultimate Beginner's Ketogenic Diet, Keto Meal Prep & Intermittent Fasting Lifestyle and Weight Loss Guide for Eating Better, Healthy Living and Feeling Good

Amy Maria Adams
Jason Brad Stephens

© **Copyright 2019 by Amy Maria Adams and Jason Brad Stephens - All rights reserved.**

The contents of this book may not be reproduced, duplicated or transmitted without direct written permission from the author.

Under no circumstances will any legal responsibility or blame be held against the publisher for any reparation, damages, or monetary loss due to the information herein, either directly or indirectly.

Legal Notice:

This book is copyright protected. This is only for personal use. You cannot amend, distribute, sell, use, quote or paraphrase any part or the content within this book without the consent of the author.

Disclaimer Notice:

Please note the information contained within this document is for educational and entertainment purposes only. Every attempt has been made to provide accurate, up to date and reliable complete information. No warranties of any kind are expressed or implied. Readers acknowledge that the author is not engaging in the rendering of legal, financial, medical or professional advice. The content of this book has been derived from various sources. Please consult a licensed professional before attempting any techniques outlined in this book.

By reading this document, the reader agrees that under no circumstances are is the author responsible for any losses, direct or indirect, which are incurred as a result of the use of information contained within this document, including, but not limited to, —errors, omissions, or inaccuracies.

About this Bundle:

Congratulations on owning *Keto Diet Complete Guide: 3 Books in 1*, and thanks for doing so.

What you are about to read is a collection of three books on the Keto Diet and Intermittent Fasting that would benefit you with your weight loss and health goals.

Book 1:
Keto Diet for Beginners

Here you will learn about the Ketogenic Diet for Beginners that helps in losing weight fast and eating better for long-term weight loss and healthy living.

Book 2:
Keto Meal Prep for Beginners

Here you will learn the best methods to save time & money for long-term weight loss, eating better and healthy living with the Keto Meal Prep.

Book 3:
Intermittent Fasting for Beginners

Here is a simple and easy-to-follow weight loss guide on how to lose weight faster, feel better and live a healthy lifestyle with Intermittent Fasting.

Thanks again for owning this book!

Let us begin with the first book in the Keto Diet bundle:

Keto Diet for Beginners

Your Ultimate & Essential Step-by-Step Ketogenic Lifestyle Guide to Losing Weight Fast and Eating Better for Long-Term Weight Loss, Healthy Living and Feeling Good

Amy Maria Adams

Table of Contents

Introduction

Chapter 1: Getting Started with the Keto Diet for Beginners

Chapter 2: Ketogenic Diet: Common Questions Answered

Chapter 3: Keto Diet: Guidelines and Food Shopping List

Chapter 4: Simple and Easy Recipes to Start (7-Day Meal Plan)

Chapter 5: The Recipes

Chapter 6: Breakfast

Chapter 7: Soups and Salads

Chapter 8: Snacks and Side Dishes

Chapter 9: Fish and Poultry

Chapter 10: Pork and Beef

Chapter 11: Desserts and Treats

Chapter 12: The 30-Day Meal Plan

Chapter 13: How to Dine Out with the Keto Diet

Chapter 14: Mistakes to avoid when on a Keto Diet

Bonus Chapter: Other Types of Keto Diet

Conclusion

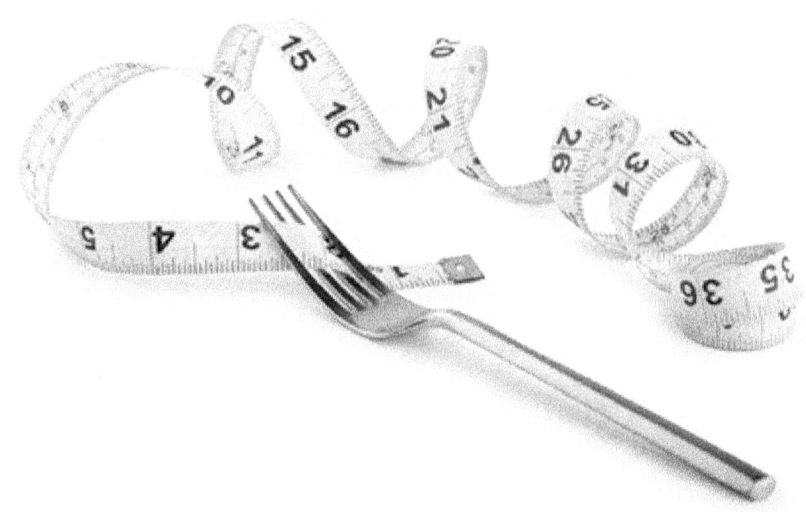

Introduction:

This book is meant to, first of all, inform you as well as serve as a guide to help you achieve that healthy lifestyle you have always desired using the ketogenic diet. The ketogenic diet is mainly natural, healthy, and at the same time, delicious. Following the ketogenic diet menu will bring about physical and mental improvements as well as help keep you energized throughout your day.

One crucial aspect of achieving success with the diet is to have a good understanding of how your body responds to food.

The keto diet was developed from fasting, which was used as a cure for epilepsy in children during the 1800s. Some believe that fasting is a cure for seizures, per the King James translation of the Bible. Mark 9:29 tells us about how Jesus cured a boy of epilepsy. When the disciples came to ask him in private why they were unable to heal (cure) the boy, Jesus stated, "this kind can come out by nothing but prayer and fasting." Notice, however, that Jesus healed the boy instantly, without recommending a fast. The most famous painting of a person with epilepsy, Raphael's *Transfiguration*, is based on this passage of scripture. The picture has two parts: the upper portion shows the transfiguration of Christ while the lower part shows the healing of the boy with epilepsy.

All kinds of diets exist—low calorie, low fat, gluten free, Weight Watchers, Atkins, South Beach, and many others. Usually, such diets entail having to starve yourself, eating uninspiring food, or being very strict about caloric intake. Many times, the challenge with these diets is that they are not nutritionally balanced and are unsatisfying. This makes them unsafe and unsustainable, meaning that you can't have a healthy lifestyle using them.

One common feature of successful diets is that they reduce foods rich in carbohydrates. Research has shown that people who eat low-fat diets and do not cut calories lose more weight than others who eat low-fat diets and also reduce calories. Also, people who eat diets low in carbohydrates usually show more improvements for important indicators like insulin and blood sugar levels, amongst many other things.

All of this depends on how your body reacts. When you eat carbohydrates, the body processes them into glucose, which is simple sugar. This leads to an increase in the levels of your blood sugar. The body then produces insulin as a way of controlling the rise in blood sugar. If you repeat this cycle over a long period, the body will naturally need to produce much more insulin at a single instance to achieve the same results.

This book will provide all you need to know to have success with the ketogenic diet. Beyond weight loss, you will learn a healthy lifestyle.

Chapter 1: Getting Started with the Keto Diet for Beginners

1.1 Definition of the Keto Diet

The ketogenic diet, also called the keto diet for short, is simply a diet that is high in fat and low in carbohydrates. It is also sometimes called low-carb, high-fat diet, or simply low-fat diet. The diet aims at reducing the intake of carbohydrates and replacing them with fat; this has many health advantages. By reducing the consumption of carbohydrates, the body is put in a metabolic state known as ketosis which is an increase in the number of ketone bodies in the blood.

When on a ketogenic diet, the body initiates a natural phenomenon in order to help us survive whenever food intake is low; this leads to efficiency in the way the body burns fat for energy. Also, fat is turned into ketones in the liver, which supplies energy for the brain; this is because the body is naturally adaptive to whatever is put into it. When there's an overload of fats and a reduction of carbohydrate intake, the body then begins to rely on ketones as its primary source of energy.

When not on a keto diet, the body relies on glucose as its source of energy, and therefore, fats are stored since they are not needed. The body chooses glucose over any other energy source because it is easy to convert. However, while on a keto diet, the body is deprived of that needed glucose, thereby forcing the body to depend on other sources of energy, in this case, fats. The ketogenic diet has recently become popular for weight loss amongst celebrities.

Who invented the keto diet?

Over the years, various dietary cures have been suggested for curing epilepsy, and many such treatments had to do with the increase or reduction of many substances like animals, vegetables, or minerals. Also, even though medical practitioners have adopted fasting as a mode of treatment for many sicknesses and ailments for more than two and a half thousand years now, fasting as a cure for seizures is not officially recognized.

The Hippocratic collection of the 5th Century BC recorded fasting as its sole treatment for epilepsy. During the fifth century BC, Hippocrates wrote about a man who had an epileptic attack. Total abstinence from food and drink was the cure for the attack.

By the early twentieth century, the ketogenic diet had been used medically as a way of replicating the biochemical impacts that a fast (or starvation) would have. The earliest scientific reports that exist about the importance of fasting in epilepsy were written by French physicians Guillaume Guelpa and Auguste Marie.

It was Dr. Russell M. Wilder, an American doctor at the Mayo Clinic, that coined the term ketogenic diet.

Dr. Wilder suggested, most likely based on the work written by Woodyatt who was also a renown medical expert, "that the advantages of fasting could be acquired if ketonemia was supplied to the body by a different means. The ketone bodies are made from fat and protein at whatever point an imbalance exists between the measures of fatty acid and sugar that are consumed in the tissues. Regardless, as has for quite some time been known, it is possible to incite ketogenesis by encouraging diets which are exceptionally rich in fat and low in carbohydrates. It is proposed in this manner, to attempt the impacts of such ketogenic diets on a set of people with epilepsy." Wilder suggested that a ketogenic diet is as effective as fasting and can be sustained for a more extended period, thereby compensating for the obvious detriments of a prolonged fast.

In a report issued the next day, he depicted the surprising improvement in the seizure control of three of his epileptic patients who were admitted to the Mayo Center to be put on the ketogenic diet. He stated that, "It is difficult to reach conclusions from the results of these set of patients who were treated with high-fat diets, yet we have here a strategy for watching the impact of ketosis on the person with epilepsy. If this is the instrument responsible for the significant impact of fasting, it might be possible to substitute for that somewhat harsh method of dietary treatment which the patient can pursue with a lesser level of inconvenience and continue at their homes as long as it seems necessary."

How the ketogenic diet works

The primary source of ketone bodies for the body is via ketogenesis. The raw materials used for this process are fatty acids in adipose tissues and amino acids that are ketogenic. Adipose tissues usually serve as a site for fat storage, and this helps in the regulation of body temperature and as an energy reserve. These stored up fatty acids can be released by a hormone known as an adipokine, which is any of the several cytokines secreted by the adipose tissue, signaling that the body has a high level of glucagon and epinephrine, and hence a low insulin level. This state connotes periods of starvation or when the glucose level in the blood is low. For the metabolism of fatty acid to lead to energy production, it must occur within the mitochondria. However, free fatty acids cannot successfully transport through the biological membrane without help; this is due to the negative electric charge they carry.

As crazy as it sounds, the way the ketogenic diet works is that to lose fat, you have eat fat; this is possible because the body is put in a state of full reliance on fats where instead of storing fats, it burns fats for energy. The body is naturally programmed to run on glucose, but while on the keto diet, carbohydrate intake is very low and therefore means little glucose will be available for the body to use. Hence, the body then changes its source of energy from glucose to ketones from fats. The body becomes a fat burning machine.

What does the ketogenic diet consist of?

A ketogenic diet is a diet that contains very low carbs and very high-fat content. It shares a lot of similarities with low-carb diets and the Atkins diet. In a keto diet, fat intake is primarily replaced with carbohydrate consumption. The aim is to obtain more calories of your daily meal from protein and fat rather than from carbs.

The drastic reduction in the intake of carbohydrates makes your body begin to adapt to such changes, therefore putting your body in a metabolic state known as ketosis. When this occurs, your body becomes an efficient "fat-burning machine." Due to a massive reduction in sugar intake, the body responds to this by converting fat into ketones, to serve as an alternative source of energy for the brain, since the brain cannot utilize fat.

Who benefits from ketogenic diets?

Being on a keto diet has numerous benefits ranging from weight loss, to reduced hunger, to improved memory retention. A ketogenic diet can help in improving health conditions such as diabetes and cardiovascular disease. Usually, any diet that aids in the excessive burning of body fat and weight reduction can reduce the risk of diabetes and certain cardiovascular diseases. And, in general, any diet that helps reduce and stabilize blood glucose, keeps blood pressure in check, and reduces triglyceride levels can prevent heart disease.

What is ketosis?

Ketosis is a state in the body in which ketone bodies in the blood are used as a primary energy source, as opposed to the state in which the glucose contained in the blood serves as the primary energy source. Usually, ketosis is said to occur when the body utilizes fat at a rapid rate, leading to the conversion of fatty acids to ketones. The state of ketosis means that the body has switched from depending on carbohydrates to burning fat for fuel. As a person lessens his or her carbohydrate intake and increases dietary fats, more fat is metabolized, and ketone bodies are created. Most fats are essential to the body and do not affect heart disease risk. Fatty acids (fat) and amino acids (protein) are necessary for living. The keto diet is a low carbohydrate, high-fat diet. A standard diet is about 50 percent carbohydrates, 35 percent fat, and 15 percent protein, but the keto diet is about 70-75 percent fat, 15-20 percent protein, and about 10 percent carbohydrates. A ketogenic diet reduces the risk factor for heart diseases like stroke, epilepsy, etc. In ketosis, your body is using ketone energy for strength instead of glucose. Entering ketosis can take a little more than three days once a person begins the keto diet. At that point, a person is using fat for energy instead of carbohydrates. The keto diet promotes fresh food like meat, fish, vegetables, and healthy fat and oils. The calorie is an essential factor in the formation of ketones. A calorie is a unit of energy. Calorie consumption dictates weight gain or loss. The macronutrient is another factor in the creation of ketones. Macronutrients are found in all foods and are measured in grams (g) on nutrition labels. Fat contains nine calories per gram while protein contains four calories per gram and carbohydrates provide four calories per gram. On a keto diet, 70-75 percent of the calories one eats should come from fat.

Ketosis is a nutritional state in which the concentration of insulin (the hormone associated with fat storage) and blood glucose is at a shallow and stable level. It is associated highly with hyperketonemia, that is, an increased level of ketone bodies within the blood. Ketones, though they can be acquired through the consumption of ketone supplements, can also be produced within the body by a process known as ketogenesis in which the glycogen stored within the body is biochemically broken down. Long-term ketosis can be a result of abstaining from food or eating a low-carb diet (keto diet). Self-induced ketosis comes with medically related benefits, e.g., curing different types of diabetes, epileptic seizure reduction, appetite control, brain injury protection, athletic performance, etc.

When glucose (glycolysis) is used as the primary source of energy, insulin levels are usually at a high level, promoting fat storage, while, in ketosis, stored-up fat is typically utilized. Because of this, ketosis is sometimes called the "fat- consuming" state.

The primary ketone bodies used as an energy source are acetoacetate and beta-hydroxybutyrate. The two hormones majorly responsible for the concentration of ketone bodies in the body are glucagon and insulin. In a normal state, most cells make use of both glucose and ketone bodies for energy.

It is important to know that ketosis is entirely different from ketoacidosis, the significant difference being in the ketone levels present in the blood. Whereas ketosis is the adapting of the body to a low-carb environment, ketoacidosis, on the other hand, is life-threatening due to the alarming concentration of glucose and ketone bodies in the blood.

Abstaining from carbohydrates to the extent of ketosis is said to have both pros and cons on a person's health. Ketosis can be stimulated by periods of starvation, or after the consumption of ketone foods and supplement.

Diagnosis of ketosis

Ketosis can be detected using a specific urine test strip, for example, Ketostix and chemstrip kits.

- Ketostix are reliable for urine testing. The chemstrip is good for at least six months.
- Chemstrip kits are the second method that can be used to check urine ketones.

How to use the Ketostix

- Collect a fresh urine sample in a dry and clean container (mix the urine specimen properly before testing.)
- Perform the test in a well-lit area (any high moisture from the air will cause the strip not to work correctly.)
- Check the expiration date on the bottle of Ketostix. A new container of Ketostix can be used for six months after the first use. Always write down the day you first open the bottle on the bottle label as using the strips beyond the expiration date may lead to poor results.
- Remove one strip from the bottle. Wipe the edges of the strip along the rim of the urine container to remove excess urine. Then turn the test strip on its side and tap it once on a piece of absorbent paper.
- Hold the strip in a vertical position and compare reagent areas to the corresponding color list on the bottle label at the specified time.
- Read your results in good light.

If your test results are inconsistent or questionable:

- Check to confirm that the bottle has not expired yet as seen on the label.
- Reconfirm your result by using another Ketostix, preferably from the

same container.

• Alternatively, you can also obtain a new bottle of strips and retest the specimen.

The closer the color is to deep purple, the more ketones are in your body. Note that the test will be difficult to interpret for anyone color-blind.

Severity of ketosis

The level of ketone bodies differs based on diet, genetic influence, exercise, metabolic adaptation, etc. Ketosis can be stimulated by staying on a ketogenic diet for more than three days; this is usually referred to as "nutritional ketosis."

It is important to note that urine measurements do not equal blood measurements, as urine concentrations are usually more hydrated and therefore lower. After staying on a ketogenic diet for a while, the concentration lost in the urine may be reduced while the metabolism still relies on ketone bodies in the blood as an energy supply. Blood tests for ketones are much more reliable; however, the test strips are costly. Urine ketone testing is notoriously unreliable.

Most urine strips only detect acetoacetate levels, while, in a severe case of ketosis, the predominant ketone body will be beta-hydroxybutyrate. At any blood level, ketones are excreted into the urine; this is quite the opposite when it comes to glucose. Ketoacidosis is a disorder that can't take place within a healthy individual who secretes insulin normally.

Controversies about ketosis

Some health experts consider abstinence from carbohydrate diets unhealthy. However, achieving a state of ketosis does not require the complete elimination of carbohydrates from the menu. Other health experts regard ketosis as a simple metabolic process that is characterized by fat-burning. Ketosis, which is usually followed by gluconeogenesis, is the particular state that worries some health experts. However, it is rare for a person in good health to reach a dangerous keto level. Individuals who suffer from the inability to secrete basal insulin are more likely to reach a life-threatening level of ketosis, eventually leading to a coma.

Signs and symptoms that can help you know if you are in ketosis

You can monitor your ketosis level using a urine or blood strip, but these are quite expensive. Alternatively, you can use specific "markers" to know if you've got it right:

- **Frequent urination** – The keto diet is a diuretic and therefore increases the rate of urine excretion. Acetoacetate, a ketone body, is usually excreted with urine.
- **Dry mouth** – the increased urination usually leads to an increase in thirst and a dry mouth. Hence, ensure you stay hydrated in order to regulate your electrolytes.
- **Mouth odor** – acetone is a ketone body that smells like an overripe fruit; it is released when we breathe. This odor gradually is reduced over the long-term.
- **Curbs hunger levels and increase energy** – a reduced hunger level usually characterizes the ketosis state.

Discomforts you may suffer during the first few weeks of being in ketosis

Your body is already well familiar with the normal process of utilizing carbohydrates as an energy source. Over time, the body secretes myriad enzymes to assist this process, but only a few enzymes associated with the breaking down of fat.

And all of a sudden, your body has to adapt to the reduction in glucose level and increase in total fat intake, which means having to build up an entirely different arsenal of enzymes. As your body initiates a state of ketosis, your body will utilize its remaining glucose reserve, breaking down glycogen in the muscles, which can cause a reduction in performance and lack of energy.

During the first week, many individuals complain of dizziness, headaches, etc. This is usually the side effects of the loss of most of your electrolytes, as ketosis increases the rate of urine excretion. These can be countered by drinking plenty of water and increasing your salt intake.

Sodium will aid with water retention and assist in replenishing flushed-out electrolytes.

What is a macro? And how to measure it?

Macros, also known as macronutrients, are fats, proteins, and carbohydrates. They play a vital role in providing our body with essential nutrients and acting as a primary energy source for our daily activities; this is what earns them the term "macro," meaning "large." We not only need them for the proper functioning of our body system, but we also need them to live.

Macro-measuring means to measure the macronutrients in your diet to ensure you're consuming the ideal daily amount of fats, proteins, and carbohydrates, although the perfect amount of each differs from individual to individual depending on certain factors like lifestyle, metabolism, and age. In other words, when measuring your macros, you will need to understand your body and what it needs. Knowing your body well may take a bit of time, but it's worth it.

How to measure macro?

They are measured in percentages, so it's not necessary to count calories; you only need to estimate what percent of each of these macros you have in your food; this makes consuming whole foods much easier since their macro content is easy to obtain. This is not the same with processed foods, whose macro-measurement is a little trickier, but not impossible. You will have to do a more in-depth label reading to find out what the food that you want to eat contains.

When macro-measuring, it is not necessary to count; you only need to measure macros. Look at everything you consume like it's a pie, and the content of each macro is a slice.

For example, your meal may contain the following; 40 percent carbs, 30 percent fats, and 30 percent protein. This is very standard and is very suitable for middle-aged individuals with an average rate of metabolism. This means that 40 percent of your daily "pie" allocation must come from carbohydrates, 30 percent from fat, and 30 percent from protein. This means that as you eat daily, you should calculate the macro percentages.

This doesn't have to be an exact science; just take mental stock of what you eat and then deduct it from your daily percentage allowance.

Thanks to the advent of the internet, you can easily use the Keto Online Calculator to calculate macros. You can access such calculator at www.ketovale.com/keto-calculator/, www.keto-calculator.ankerl.com/, www.ketokarma.com/keto-calculator and many websites available online. These websites take your body type and activity level into consideration, so you can rest assured that they're quite correct.

Understand your body

Your sex and age play a minor role in determining your exact macro requirements. Your body type is the primary factor that affects and determines your macro requirements. You have to understand your metabolism, which is your physiological self, to achieve accurate macro measurements. In general, we have three body types. They include:

• **Ectomorph** – this body type is slender, with a small bone structure, and gaining weight and muscle mass can be difficult. An individual in this category will require a macro constituent of 50-60 percent carbs, 30-40 percent protein, and 20-30 percent fat.

• **Mesomorph** – this body type is naturally strong and muscular, with broad shoulders and very dense bones. Gaining or losing weight is moderately easy, while gaining muscle mass is very easy. Individuals in this category will require a macro constituent of 40-50 percent carbs, 35-45 percent protein, and 25-35 percent fat.

• **Endomorphs** – this body type is stocky, involving a round body and shorter limbs. Gaining muscle mass is very easy, but losing weight is extremely hard. Individuals in this category will require a macro constituent of 20-30 percent carbs, 30-40 percent fat, and 50-60 percent protein.

Even after understanding how your body functions, you will still have to adjust your macros to suit your goals and daily activity level. In general, if your goal is to burn fat and gain muscle, your protein percentage should be the highest. Your carb intake should be the lowest, and your fat intake should remain moderate.

1.2 Benefits of keto diets

The ketogenic diet differs from other diets in the sense that many of those diets offer weight loss as their main advantage. The ketogenic diet comes with a large number of benefits because of the way it alters the chemical composition of the body. The keto diet leads to an increase in the production of ketones, as well as a dependence on ketones for the daily maintenance of the body. The body is more efficient when it depends on ketones as fuel. Amongst the many advantages of the ketogenic diet, a few will be discussed below:

- **Weight loss** – because of its low carbohydrate content, the ketogenic diet brings about a breaking down of body fat into ketones and allows the body to depend mainly on ketones rather than glucose. In other words, the fat stored up in the body will be used as a source of energy. When an individual is on a keto diet, insulin, which is the fat-storing hormone level, drops massively, turning the body into a fat-consuming machine since fat storage is prevented. Scientifically, on long-term analysis, a regularly practiced ketogenic diet has proven to show better results as compared to low-fat and high-carb diets; cholesterol is produced from the conversion of excess glucose in the diet. Ketogenic diets generally have an improved feeling of satiety, hence leading to an overall reduction in food intake. This allows for reduced calorie intake without necessarily causing ravenous hunger.

- **Reversion of nephropathy** – nephropathy is one of the complications associated with individuals who have uncontrolled diabetes. Studies have shown that keto diets aid the reversing of diabetic nephropathy by increasing the level of 3-beta-hydroxybutyric acid in the blood, which leads to the subsequent reduction in the metabolism of glucose in some tissues within the body, for example, the kidneys. In a study performed by Poplawski et al., during one week of administering the ketogenic diets to rats, the glucose level in the blood normalized. Within two months, the albumin/creatinine ratio was also standardized, and diabetic nephropathy was completely reversed. This is associated with the expression of genes induced by oxidation and various forms of stress being normalized. In a human, the ketogenic diet causes a decrease in the level of creatinine as compared to the consumption of low-calorie foods, which show an increase in the level of creatinine. Ketones can serve as an alternative source of energy.

• **Boost brain health** – the brain, unlike the muscles, cannot utilize fat as a source of energy; therefore, the brain is heavily dependent on glucose. The brain, however, can utilize ketones. The liver uses fatty acid to produce ketones in situations where glucose and insulin levels are low. Ketones are usually produced in little amounts when one hasn't eaten for long hours, for example, after a full night's sleep. However, the liver's production of ketones increases during periods of fasting, starvation, or when the level of carb intake is below 50 g per day. When the consumption of carbs is minimized, ketones can cater for up to 70 percent of the brain's needs. Although most of the brain can utilize ketones, some parts depend solely on glucose for their functionality. When one is on a low-carb diet, some of this glucose can be provided for by the small intake of carbs. The body, however, synthesizes most of the glucose requirements in a process known as gluconeogenesis. In this metabolic process, the liver produces glucose for the brain to utilize; it uses amino acids as its raw material. The liver can also produce glucose from glycerol; this is the backbone that connects fatty acids in triglyceride molecules—the body's form of storing fat. Staying on a ketogenic diet has been proven to be effective against Parkinson's disease as well. It is most likely that certain features associated with remaining on a ketogenic diet, such as an increase in brain sharpness, mental clarity, and less frequent migraines are related to the controlled level of sugar in the blood serum and change of energy source for the brain, which helps improve memory.

• **Increase in the levels of HDL cholesterol** – whenever people hear about an increase in the level of cholesterol, there is usually a panic, and this is because many are not well informed that there are two types of cholesterol (the HDL and the LDL). The HDL is the one that is more needed because it carries cholesterol from the body to the liver (the liver is where it can be reused or excreted.) Conversely, the LDL transports cholesterol from the liver to all parts of the body.

- **Reduction of epileptic seizures** – seizures are a complication associated with epilepsy. It usually manifests as continuous jerking movements and fainting; it occurs mostly in children. Epilepsy is tough to treat. There are several types of seizures. Although many effective anti-seizure medications exist, these drugs are usually ineffective in at least 30 percent of epilepsy patients. This type of epilepsy is known as "unresponsive to medication." The ketogenic diet, developed by Dr. Russell Wilder in 1921, supplies the body with about 90 percent of calories from fat and is effective in treating drug-resistant epilepsy in children, as it has been said to imitate the important effects that starvation has on seizures. The particular mechanism, however, remains unknown, but it is believed to help in increasing the stability of neurons and regulation of mitochondrial enzymes.

- **Beneficial for individuals with Alzheimer's disease** – ketogenic diets provide benefits to people with Alzheimer's disease. Alzheimer's is a gradually advancing disease in which the brain develops tangles that result in loss of memory. Many researchers believe that it should be classified as "type 3" diabetes because the brain cells develop insulin resistance and lack the ability to utilize glucose properly, causing inflammation. Health experts claim that Alzheimer's disease has certain common features with epilepsy, for example, overexcitement of the brain cells that leads to seizures. It has been suggested that ketogenic diets may be an effective method of fueling brain cells affected by Alzheimer's disease. One hypothesis is that ketone bodies protect the cells of the brain by limiting the level of reactive oxygen species which are by-products of metabolism that may cause inflammation. Another hypothesis states that the lethal proteins that accumulate in the brains of individuals with Alzheimer's disease can be reduced by a diet that contains a high amount of fat.

- **Battling cancer** – cancerous cells express a metabolism that is different from the metabolism of healthy cells. They are usually characterized by rapid increase in glucose utilization. This is due to the many insulin receptors in them, causing them to thrive in an environment that has high levels of both insulin and blood sugar, usually caused by mutations and mitochondrial dysfunction. Cancerous cells, unlike healthy cells, cannot effectively utilize ketone bodies as an energy source. Also, ketone bodies restrain the proliferation of tumor cells, and they can provide energy for healthy cells without feeding the tumor cells. Ketogenic diets, however, can only be helpful against some types of cancer.

- **Boosts energy levels and improves sleep** – after staying on a ketogenic diet for about four to five days, most individuals experience an increase in energy levels and a general lack of interest in carbohydrate diets; this is as a result of a readily available energy source and the insulin level being stabilized in body and brain tissues. When placed on a low-carb diet, the body can only store so much glycogen, and as a result, constant refueling is necessary to maintain energy levels. However, your body already has as alternative fat storage to utilize; this means that ketosis is a source of fuel to the body that can never be exhausted and you'll find that you have energy throughout the day. The mechanism of sleep improvement remains a mystery. However, studies have shown that staying on a ketogenic diet helps improve sleep by reducing REM and increasing slow-wave sleep patterns. This is most likely related to the biochemical shifts associated with the brain now depending on ketone bodies as an alternate energy source and other body tissues breaking down fat. However, during the first few weeks of staying on a ketogenic diet (the adjustment period), you may experience particular difficulties in staying asleep and insomnia. This will wane with time as your body becomes accustomed to ketosis and to consuming stored-up fat. And then you'll find that you feel more relaxed, can sleep deeply for more hours, and feel rested when you wake.

- **Aids kidney functions** – kidney stones and gout are mostly caused by an increase in uric acid, phosphate, and calcium levels. This is as a result of obesity, dehydration, consumption of sugar (especially fructose), and alcohol consumption. Uric acid levels can be temporarily increased by ketogenic diets, especially when a person is dehydrated, though its level decreases over time. Uric acid levels increase within the same time frame as ketone bodies, but after a period of four to six weeks, uric acid levels begin to decrease despite ketone levels staying up. Hence, the individual might have a low uric acid level despite being in a state of nutritional ketosis.
- **Helping women's health** – polycystic ovary syndrome (PCOS) can be effectively treated with low-carbohydrate diets which help to stop specific symptoms such as obesity, infrequent menstrual periods, and acne. Keto diets also help in keeping the level of sugar in the blood serum deficient and stabilized. They also help to maintain the level of other hormones, and especially in women, this has a lot of benefits in a wide variety of metabolic pathways associated with insulin.
- **Helps battle type 2 diabetes** – individuals that suffer from type 2 diabetes exhibit excessive insulin production. Because keto diets are low-carb and hence remove sugar from the food, they assist in the reduction of the HbA1c count. That can, therefore, help reverse type 2 diabetes. Ketogenic diets also help in reversing nephrology, provide cardiac benefits, assist with weight loss, and improve lipid profiles.
- **Helps boost gastrointestinal health and liver health** – it is common knowledge that grain-based foods, nightshade vegetables (such as tomatoes, potatoes, etc.), and sugar-filled foods increase the chances of heartburn and acid reflux. It is, therefore, of little surprise that maintaining a low-carb diet helps improve these symptoms, confronting the problems of autoimmune responses and inflammation. With regards to this, changes in diet alter the total human gut microbiome (you are what you eat). A variation in the microbiome substantially reduces most gastrointestinal problems as a result of staying on the ketogenic diet.

Studies have shown that carbs in the diet are highly associated with gallstones as they are the main ingredients that cause them. As a countereffect, eating an appropriate amount of fat when carb intake is down assists in the clearing out of the gallbladder and improves functionality, thus reducing the chances of gallstones forming. Fat accumulating in the liver is related to prediabetes and type 2 diabetes; in very extreme cases, fatty liver disease can be very lethal to the liver. This condition is usually tested using a blood test to measure the level of liver enzymes.

- **Decreases inflammation** – ketogenic diets are highly anti-inflammatory and help in improving a lot of health problems. The anti-inflammatory properties of ketogenic diets, or a reduction in caloric intake, may be linked to retardation of the hormone responsible for inflammation. In other words, the main ingredients responsible for most inflammatory diseases are repressed by ketone bodies made from a ketogenic diet. Thus, its effect on acne, psoriasis, eczema, arthritis, and other inflammation-associated diseases is reasonably significant enough to attract more research attention. It is, therefore, very possible to improve a whole host of conditions through nutritional ketosis.

- **Helps in appetite control** – when staying on a low-carb diet, you'll find that you don't feel hungry as often as before; you don't develop random cravings that make you go on an excessive snacking spree and cause you to eat bad things. Many individuals that stay on a ketogenic diet find it easier to perform intermittent fasting, where you're feeding not as consistently as before, and you only get to eat at certain set periods of the day. Controlling the sugar level in the blood can help with curbing such cravings and uncontrollable appetites.

This book will help every newbie understand the keto diet; there are recipes within the book to try out which will improve your health and well-being.

1.3

One of the ways you can find out how much you know, do not know or need to know about the keto diet as a beginner and is to take online tests. That's a good way of checking your knowledge base (if it's sound enough) and there are many websites where you can take such tests. You can take tests at "Completely Keto" at http://completelyketo.com or "Bhu Foods" at http://bhufoods.com

Your Quick Start Action Step:

Create some time before the end of the day to take the test at any of the websites listed above and take the tests.

None of the tests should take more than 15 to 20 minutes.

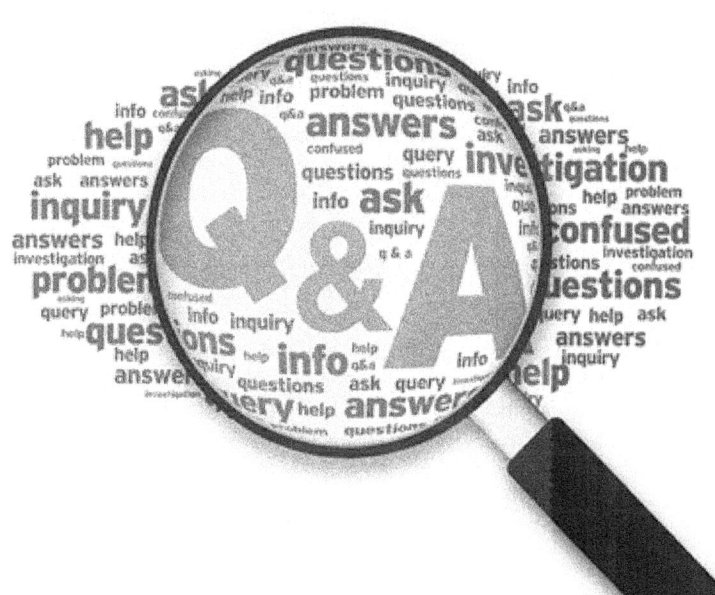

Chapter 2: The Ketogenic Diet – Common Questions Answered

2.1 Is the ketogenic diet safe?

It is normal that whenever a new diet hits the scene, there's always information that talks about its negative impacts on your health. However, what is the case with the keto diet? The keto diet has undergone scientific tests and analysis and has been recommended by great medical institutions globally. It has been proven to be safe; however, this depends on the activity level and condition of the individual. But on a general scale, it is entirely safe. It is helpful for achieving a healthy lifestyle and not just a miracle cure.

2.2 Does the ketogenic diet work?

The ketogenic diet has been in use for a very long time; it became more pronounced in the 1920s and since then has been used repeatedly on different individuals. The keto diet started as a cure for epileptic children, with many of them being completely cured. The ketogenic diet has been proven to work for many conditions starting from weight loss to heart disease. Its impact on weight loss has been debated as a short-term impact; some patients apparently regain weight after about a year or two. But this is highly debatable.

2.3 Does the ketogenic diet work for the long-term?

It is highly debatable whether the use of ketogenic diets for weight loss works for the long-term; however, it is not medically or scientifically proven otherwise. Using weight loss for other diseases works, for example, for people with diabetes, and the cure is long-term. The same thing applies to high-blood pressure if they are able to follow through with the diet successfully.

2.4 Does the ketogenic diet affect weight loss?

The answer is yes. The ketogenic diet is gaining popularity again not precisely because of its benefits for other diseases but because of its use for weight loss. The ketogenic diet is beneficial for weight loss because of the dramatic reduction in the intake of carbohydrates, forcing the body to burn fat as its source of energy rather than glucose from carbohydrates. It also reduces appetite, which also contributes to weight loss. By affecting appetite, it reduces individuals' cravings for sugar.

2.5 How does a ketogenic diet affect cholesterol?

It is a common misconception that since ketogenic diets are high in fat content, they lead to an increase in cholesterol levels in the body. However, this is not true. Much scientific research has shown that low-carb diets help in optimizing the cholesterol level in the body. Many are unaware that there is good cholesterol and bad cholesterol. HDL cholesterol is the one known as "the good cholesterol." It collects all cholesterol that is not in use within the body and takes it to the liver, where it is either recycled or destroyed. The ketogenic diet causes a reduction in LDL, "the bad cholesterol," which is responsible for some cardiovascular diseases in adults.

2.6 What is the "keto flu" and how do you minimize it?

Starting a keto diet can be very strange. You have a lot to look forward to including a lot of weight loss and a lot of anticipated internal changes that your body is bound to undergo. However, keto flu is something else that might also come along when starting a keto diet. Your body may experience keto flu during the initial stages of being on a keto diet. Usually, the body gets a little weak before it finally starts getting stronger. The extent to which your body suffers usually depends largely on your previous diet as it determines the shock your system will undergo from your new diet pattern; the effect of that shock is what you will begin to experience.

Once you start a keto diet, some symptoms are sure markers of having the keto flu. They include:

- Headaches

- A cough

- Fatigue

- Irritability

- Nausea

These symptoms are usually indications that your body needs to adjust to the changes in your diet pattern and adapt to what you're putting it through. Having these symptoms is not enjoyable, and it sucks; they can leave you discouraged and make you wonder whether it is worth the pain and discomfort. However, these symptoms will eventually fade away as your body approaches ketosis. These symptoms are just your body reacting to carb deprivation, but over time, these symptoms will go just as quickly as they came.

A ketogenic diet contains a very low-carb content, and therefore your body tries to adapt to the low intake of carbs since you have been consuming a large amount of carbs your whole life up to this point. Staying away from carbs will tend to come as a shock to your body, but very soon your body will recover and continues on the path to good health. When suffering from the keto flu, you may start to consider eating more carbs to make the pain and discomfort go away, but do not listen to this temptation; endure for a couple of days, and everything will go back to normal.

How to minimize the flu?

Once on a keto diet, one of the numerous changes your body will undergo is a loss of body fluids and electrolytes in the form of sodium, potassium, and magnesium. Electrolytes are vital to the proper functioning of your body as they play a significant role in determining the amount of water in your body and how effectively your muscles perform their task. Carbs usually help with water retention within the body, ensuring there is no excessive loss of electrolytes. When staying on a keto diet, you will begin to lose a lot of body fluids, and since most electrolytes are dissolved in these fluids as a solvent, it is natural that you will lose some of them. Also, since your body is going to be consuming a lot of stored-up body fat, and your body cells will begin to replace these fats with water, it is essential to stay hydrated. It is also necessary to add a lot of salt to your daily meal by eating foods that have a high sodium content. If your electrolyte consumption is high, then you'll be just fine.

How long will it take for my body to adjust?

When on a regular diet, your body is, necessarily, sugar dependent but when on a keto diet, your body becomes fat dependent. This kind of change usually has a drastic effect on the body, but time is all your body requires. The adjustment period differs with individuals. However, on average, it takes more than a week to finally reach the ketosis stage; for some, it occurs faster than that. It all depends on how your body reacts to the effect of such changes; this is the time your body begins to shed some fat. It is essential to note that even when your body has reached the ketosis stage, that doesn't mean it will stay in it when you begin to eat carbs again. Some individuals can get away with it; others can't. It is just safer to adhere strictly to your diet.

2.7 How many carbs can I eat on the keto diet?

The amount of carbs every individual needs is dependent on a couple of things. Generally, eating less carbs has more impact. It will speed weight loss and reduce appetite and hunger. Someone with type 2 diabetes should eat fewer carbohydrates; it will improve insulin resistance. The truth is that many people find a diet that is very low in carbs somewhat too challenging and restrictive.

2.8 How much protein should I eat on the keto diet?

When on a keto diet, it is essential to eat a lot of protein. However, if you eat too much of it, this will lower your ketone levels; if you eat too little, it leads to you losing excess muscle. So you should be at the midpoint in that sense. For someone that is sedentary, that is, you do a whole lot of sitting during the day, you should eat around 0.6 grams and 0.8 grams of protein for every pound of lean body mass. If you are someone who has an active day, you should eat between 0.8 grams and one gram of protein for every pound of lean body mass. If you want to gain some muscle, you should eat about one gram and 1.2 grams of protein for every pound of lean body mass. You don't need more protein than that.

2.9 What ketogenic diet is best?

In selecting the best diet, there are some things to consider. If you're someone who rarely engages in highly intense exercise and wants to lose weight, you should stick to the standard keto diet. If you add more carbohydrates, you will only be slowing down your progress and prolong how long it takes to reach ketosis, unlike those who don't add carbs. For people who engage in intense exercise regularly, then the cyclical keto diet and the targeted keto diet might be right for you. If you're someone who has only started intense workouts regularly within the last year, you should try out the targeted keto diet and see if you notice a decrease in performance while you're on the standard keto diet. When it comes to figuring out the best type of keto diet for you, it is important that you experiment. There are no individuals that are the same; you must find out what works for you best. It is important also to note that if you're not doing intense exercise regularly, then you should stay on the standard keto diet. Usually, most people do not need anything more than the standard keto diet.

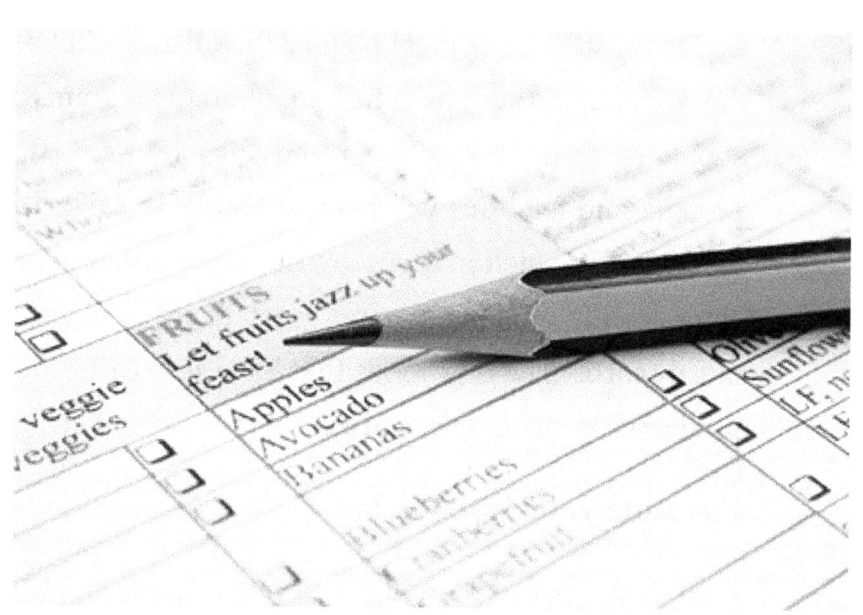

Chapter 3: Keto Diet – Guidelines and Food Shopping List

3.1 Guidelines for the ketogenic diet

Find out what you need to eat and avoid while on the diet

To follow a keto diet meal plan or food list, you'll be reducing carbs on a diet. You should start by eating about 20 to 30 grams of carbs per day. You should do some research and find out food items that are mostly carbs, protein, and fats; this will help you make the right choices. Examples of foods that are high in carbs are not just limited to pasta, bread, cookies, chips, candy, and ice cream. Most fruits and vegetables also contain mostly carbs. The only foods that have zero carbs are meat (protein) and pure fats like oil and margarine.

Examine your love for fat

Keto diets involve a whole lot of fats, so you must love them. Many are scared of eating fats because they have been told it will kill them. Before starting the keto diet, begin by adjusting your daily food intake to accommodate high fats; you can substitute green vegetables for fries or order a burger on lettuce leaves. Rather than rice or potatoes, you can eat a non-starchy vegetable. Cook with more oil. Slowly introduce fats into your meals and reduce the carb content. The keto diet won't work for you if you're the type that is scared of fats.

Sharpen your cooking abilities

You need to sharpen your cooking skills as high-carb processed foods are a no-go area while on a diet. You must learn how to make fresh meals. You can have a look at the sample recipes in the later chapters of this book, and you'll fall in love with them. Check out recipes you know you will like online as well. By doing this, you will lessen the chances of having to revert to carbs.

Try keto-friendly drinks

You should try bulletproof coffee. It's one of the greatest warm keto beverages. It's made by just mixing butter and coconut oil with your coffee. This drink reduces hunger levels, thereby allowing you extra time to plan your next meal properly.

A note of caution: if you have heart disease, then you might want to avoid this drink. For safety's sake, you should ask your doctor if it is safe for you.

Speak with your family about your goals on the diet

Clearly state your plan. You will not be able to eat all meals with them, so you will have to make your meals yourself. Sometimes, there might be an objection. Explain that you have adequately researched the diet, have found it to be safe, and want to try this out.

Clean out your pantry

When you decide to go on the keto diet, one of the first things to do is to discard everything that is anti-keto. Keeping tempting but unhealthy foods around your home can be the biggest cause of failure for your keto diet. Hence, to achieve success, you must reduce such temptations to a bearable minimum. Unless you are very strong-willed, you shouldn't keep tempting foods such as desserts, loaves of bread very high in sugar, and other anti-keto snacks around you.

If you're the kind of person who lives with others, ensure you inform your housemates and family members, as well as other people you live with, and warn them before throwing anything out of the house. If some food items must be hidden (that is, if they're not yours and can't be thrown out), you all should agree about a good place where they can be out of sight. Doing this will make it clear to those you live with that you are pretty serious about your new diet, and will ultimately result in a great experience for you at home. It is normal for people to want to tempt you when you start a new diet, but eventually, as time passes, they'll stop.

Some of the things you should keep away include;

Sugary foods and drinks: You need to get rid of all processed sugar, fruit juices, desserts, pastries, fountain drinks, milk, milk chocolate, candy bars, etc.

Fruits: Get rid of all fruits that have a high-carb content; this includes apples, mangoes, dates, bananas, and grapes. You must ensure you rid yourself of all dried fruits like raisins, too. Dried fruits usually have as much sugar as regular fruits, but they're even more concentrated which makes it easy to consume a whole lot of sugar in small servings. For instance, a cup of raisins contains 100 grams of carbohydrates; meanwhile, a cup of grapes contains about 15 grams of carbs.

Starches and grains: You should get rid of all types of cereal, rice, corn, rolls, pasta, wraps, oats, bread, quinoa, bagels, flour, potatoes, and croissants.

Processed polyunsaturated fats and oils: Get rid of most seed oils. Seed oils to eliminate include safflower, corn oil, grapeseed, sunflower, and canola. Also, get rid of trans fats like margarine and shortening—anything that reads "hydrogenated," even if it's partial. The kind of oils you should keep at home are coconut oil, olive oil, avocado oil, and extra-virgin olive oil. These are the keto-friendly ones.

Legumes: You should also get rid of beans, lentils, and peas. They are highly concentrated with carbs. A typical one-cup serving of beans contains three times more carbs than you should consume in a day.

Don't miss the point: you are meant to get rid of all keto-unfriendly food items, but these foods are still good for others. Hence, you shouldn't throw them into the trash can; other people can eat them. Look for people around you to whom you can donate them. Your pantry should look empty after you clean it out; this is because most of the food items that can be stored for the long-term are usually high in carbs and usually contain unhealthy preservatives and additives.

Kitchen utensils to use

Having the right low-carb kitchen gadgets can make life a little easier and your diet more successful. You shouldn't waste money on kitchen utensils that are unnecessary. Some of them might be things you have in your kitchen already.

• Kitchen Scales

Kitchen scales are important for measuring out menu sizes for beginners. Without kitchen scales, it will be hard to know the macronutrient size of your food since you can't say how much you eat. The keto diet requires that you cook by weight. It is entirely accurate, and there is no room for error. Recipe failures are sometimes because people cook by volume (that is, using cups). They usually fill their cups too firmly or too loosely, thereby leading to adding too much or too little of an ingredient or food item, making the recipe a disaster. Start using electronic scales and save yourself some trouble. You can easily switch between ounces or grams, depending on what you want. Making use of scales also reduces your washing up. Zero the scales, add your first food item, zero the scales again, and then add your second item, etc.

• Slow Cooker

This is perfect for making recipes while you're on the go. Set it before you leave and forget it!

The slow cooker is a great utensil. It makes life easier. If you know you have a crazy day ahead and won't be home until late after sports and other activities are finished, always put on the slow cooker. By the time you walk in the door, dinner will already be waiting.

• Frying Pan/Skillet

Try to buy one with a heavy base so the heat is well distributed and steady. You will notice the difference.

One utensil to love is the electric frying pan. If you want to cook a big breakfast for a family of five, you have to squeeze in bacon, eggs, greens, and tomatoes. That is the way to conveniently cook a full meal in one go.

The eggs cook perfectly with the lid on, the bacon doesn't dry up, and they all remain warm if you're still in the shower when breakfast is ready. No more messing up two frying pans or keeping things warm in the oven.

• Spiralizers (Handheld, Benchtop)

Vegetable noodles are popular and are a better/healthier substitute for pasta.

Handheld spiralizers are very easy to take along on holiday with you but can be a little slower to use, and you need to keep your little fingers away from the exposed sharp blades lest they cut you.

The benchtop spiralizer is the fast one. Plus, it's fun for the children to use. It is very safe and washes easily. It comes with different three blades to create varied sized ribbons of "pasta" or noodles.

• Stick Blender

I recommend buying a stick blender with multiple attachment options. You can use the mini processor to grind nuts and almonds, and the whisk to whip cream.

• Food Processor

This is another kitchen utensil that you must have for pureeing and chopping.

It can be used for grating/shredding carrots for making low-carb carrot cake, and it's great for cheese, because buying pre-grated/shredded cheese will cost you a whole lot more. You can also use it for making a flourless orange cake.

• **Measuring Cups And Spoons**

These are important for the same reason as the kitchen scale. If you want to know exactly what your servings are, measuring cups and spoons help you to do this. Also, measuring correctly enables you to achieve better-tasting recipes!

• **Mixing Bowls, Various Sizes**

You can choose to buy stackable mixing bowls to save space in your cupboards. If you can find those with lids, they can also be used for storage in the fridge.

• **Baking Trays, Cake Pans**

Loose-bottom cake pans can be used for chocolate heaven cake and lemon coconut cake to ensure it cooks evenly.

• **Roasting Pan**

One great meal you can always have is roasted meat and vegetables. It can be prepared on a regular basis.

You can put two roasting pans in the oven every time. One for the vegetables and meat, and another for preparing your grain-free granola.

• **Parchment Paper, Non-Stick Baking Sheets/Silicone Mat**

These are important for preparing some recipes like the Fat head pizza as well as to line cake pans.

Ensure you have these so you don't difficulties cleaning up when you're done cooking or baking.

• Knives

You should have a good solid knife set in your kitchen. They can make all the difference.

They'll make your cooking safer, faster, and easier.

• Mortar And Pestle

You will be doing some grinding. You can use a mortar and pestle to grind granulated sweetener in case you run out.

A powdered sweetener is an essential ingredient for making sugar-free chocolate shells; also, it is easier to add it to fat bombs or fudge.

• Waffle Maker And Coffee Maker

These are not so important, but can make your keto life nicer.

• Egg Cooker

If you love eating eggs, then you should have one of these. They can poach or boil many eggs at a time.

Having an egg cooker is a good choice if you have to cook some boiled eggs for school lunches for the next day. This will save you from having to go to the grocery store numerous times.

• Food-Prep Bowls With Covers, And Storage Containers

You will need to have storage containers. You will need as many as you can use to keep a couple of meals in the fridge, including any leftovers.

It's also good to have a range of tiny containers to put leftovers in so you can add them to school lunchboxes in the morning. Nothing should go to waste.

- **Kids' Lunchboxes**

If you want to be a real food family who has ditched the junk food and processed food, you'll need a decent lunchbox.

- **Silicon Cupcake Cases**

These are awesome for cooking and perfect for lunchboxes.

Not only are these great for making low-carb cupcakes, but they are also handy for serving berries in a lunchbox or little cheese cubes, setting mini Jell-Os, or making fat bombs. You should have silicon cupcake cases in a variety of shapes.

- **Ice-Cream Makers**

For regular ice cream, it is not essential to have an ice-cream maker. But having an ice-cream maker makes a lovely, light, and fluffy scoop.

Shopping list

Below is a comprehensive list of what a shopping list should include; the carb content for each food item is also mentioned to help you make an informed decision. Eating less carbs can have amazing medical benefits. It has been proven to diminish general hunger levels, which will, in turn, lead to dramatic weight loss without having to keep checking your calorie intake.

About 23 studies have shown that low-carb diets can cause up to two times more weight loss than low-fat diets. Eating low-carb doesn't need to be technical.

To get thinner and improve your health, just make sure your diet contains natural foods that are low in carbs. Listed below are some low-carb foods that should be found on your keto shopping list, all of which are nutritious, healthy, and unimaginably delicious.

The amount of carbs for a standard serving, and the number of carbs in a 100-gram serving, are listed toward the end of each segment.

In any case, remember that some of these foods have very high fiber content, which may reduce the absorbable net carb.

Meats and Eggs

Eggs, and a wide range of beef, are near zero carbs. Organ meats are a peculiar case. For example, liver contains about five percent carbs.

• **Eggs (almost zero)**

Eggs are some of the most beneficial and nutritional foods on earth. They contain different nutrients—including some that are essential for your mind— and can enhance the health of your eyes. Eggs have almost zero carbs.

• **Beef (zero)**

Beef is profoundly satisfying and full of essential nutrients like iron and vitamin B12. There are many diverse kinds of beef, from ground beef to ribeye steak to hamburger. Beef contains zero carbs.

• **Lamb (zero)**

Like beef, lamb contains numerous advantageous nutrients, including iron and vitamin B12. Lamb is regularly grass-nourished, and will, in general, be high in the essential fatty acid conjugated linoleic acid (CLA). Lamb has zero carbs.

• **Chicken (zero)**

Chicken is among the world's most common meats. It's high in numerous helpful nutrients and a fantastic source of protein. In case you're on a low-carb diet, it might be a good decision to go for fattier cuts like wings and thighs. Chicken has zero carbs.

- **Pork, including Bacon (usually zero)**

Pork is another tasty kind of meat, and bacon is the most loved protein for numerous low-carb dieters. Bacon is processed meat, and consequently might not be so healthy. Be that as it may, it's generally acceptable to eat reasonable amounts of bacon on a low-carb diet.

Endeavor to purchase your bacon locally, without artificial additives, and don't burn it while cooking. It usually contains zero carbs; however, check the label and maintain a strategic distance from bacon that is treated with sugar.

- **Jerky (usually zero)**

Jerky is meat that has been processed into smaller strips and dried. As long as it doesn't contain added sugar or artificial additives, jerky can be an ideal low-carb snack food.

It is important you note that a lot of the jerky available at many stores is highly processed and therefore unhealthy. Your best option is to make your own.

Depending on the type, if it's mainly meat plus seasoning, it ought to be near zero carbs.

Other examples of low-carb meats include;

Turkey

Buffalo

Venison

Seafood

Fish and different kinds of seafood are usually extraordinarily nutritious and healthy. They're exceptionally high in B12, iodine, and omega-3 fatty acids—all nutrients which numerous individuals don't get enough of. Like beef, a wide range of fish and seafood contains almost no carbs.

• Salmon (zero)

Salmon is a standout amongst the most popular sorts of fish among health-conscious people—for obviously good reasons. It's a fatty fish, which implies that it contains large measures of heart-healthy fats, particularly omega-3 fatty acids. Salmon is additionally packed with vitamin B12, iodine, and a good amount of vitamin D3. It contains zero carbs.

• Trout (zero)

Like salmon, trout is a fatty fish that is stacked with omega-3 fatty acids and other essential vitamins. It has zero carbs.

• Sardines (zero)

Sardines are small, oily fish that are, for the most part, eaten whole, including their bones. Sardines are among the most nutrient-filled foods on earth and contain pretty much every vitamin that your body needs. They contain zero carbs.

• Shellfish (4-5% carbs)

It's shameful that shellfish almost never makes it onto some individuals' everyday menus as they're one of the world's most nutritious food. They rank near organ meats in their nutrient concentration and are low in carbs. They usually contain four to five grams of carbs per 100 grams of shellfish.

Other Low-Carb Fish and Seafood

Shrimp

Catfish

Haddock

Lobster

Herring

Cod

Vegetables

Most vegetables contain low carbs. Leafy greens and cruciferous vegetables have unusually low amounts, and the more substantial part of their carbs comprise of fiber. Then again, starchy root vegetables like potatoes and sweet potatoes are high in carbs.

Broccoli (7%)

Broccoli is a delicious cruciferous vegetable that can be eaten both raw and cooked. It's rich in vitamin C, vitamin K, and fiber and contains strong anti-cancer plant compounds. It contains six grams of carbs per cup, or seven grams for every 100 grams.

Tomatoes (4%)

Tomatoes are fruits or berries that are typically eaten as vegetables. They're high in potassium and vitamin C. There are seven grams of carb in an average large tomato or four grams for every 100 grams.

Onions (9%)

Onions are among the most delicious plants on earth and add incredible flavor to your meals. They're high in fiber, cancer prevention agents, and different inflammatory compounds. There are nine grams of carbs for every 100 grams.

Brussels Sprouts (7%)

Brussels grows exceptionally nutritious vegetables, closely related with broccoli and kale. They're high in vitamins C and K and contain various valuable plant compounds. There are about six grams of carbs for every half cup, or seven grams for every 100 grams.

Cauliflower (5%)

Cauliflower is a delicious and flexible vegetable that can be utilized to make different intriguing dishes in your kitchen. It's high in folate, vitamin C, and vitamin K. It contains five grams of carbs for each cup and five grams for every 100 grams.

Kale (10%)

Kale is a favorite vegetable among health-conscious people, offering various medical advantages.

It's stacked with fiber, vitamins C and K, and also carotene cancer prevention agents. It contains seven grams of carbs per cup, or 10 grams for every 100 grams.

Eggplant (6%)

Eggplant is another organic product that is generally devoured as a vegetable. It has many exciting uses and is high in fiber. It contains five grams of carbs cup, or six grams for every 100 grams.

Cucumber (4%)

Cucumber is a common vegetable with a gentle flavor. It is generally comprised of water, with a little measure of vitamin K. It contains two grams of carbs for every half cup, or four grams for every 100 grams.

Bell Peppers (6%)

Bell peppers are well known natural products/vegetables with an unmistakable and fulfilling taste. They're high in fiber, vitamin C, and carotene cancer prevention agents. They contains nine grams of carbs for every cup, or six grams for every 100 grams.

Asparagus (2%)

Asparagus is a very delicious spring vegetable. It's high in fiber, vitamin C, folate, vitamin K, and carotene cancer prevention agents. Also, it's high in protein, contrasted with general vegetables. It contains three grams of carbs for every cup, or two grams for every 100 grams.

Green Beans (7%)

Green beans are legumes, yet they're usually eaten similarly as vegetables. Calorie by calorie, they're, to a significant degree, high in numerous nutrients, including vitamin C, protein, fiber, vitamin K, magnesium, and potassium. They contain eight grams of carbs for every cup, or seven grams for every 100 grams.

Mushrooms (3%)

Even though they're not plants, edible mushrooms are regularly grouped as vegetables. They contain decent measures of potassium and are highly concentrated in some B vitamins. They contain three grams of carbs for every glass, and three grams for every 100 grams (white mushrooms).

Other Low-Carb Vegetables

Celery

Spinach

Zucchini

Swiss chard

Cabbage

Except for starchy root vegetables, almost all vegetables have low-carb content. That is the reason you can eat a whole lot of them without going beyond your carb limit.

Fruits

Even though fruits are generally believed to be healthy, this is a bit controversial for those on a low-carb diet.

That is because most fruits will, in general, be high in carbs, as opposed to vegetables.

Depending on what amount of carbs you are planning to eat, you may need to confine your fruit intake to one to two pieces per day. However, this is not the case for fatty fruits like olives or avocados. Low-sugar fruits, for example, strawberries, are another excellent choice.

Avocado (8.5%)

The avocado is quite a unique kind of fruit. Rather than being high in carbs, it contains solid fats. Avocados are, to a significant degree, high in fiber and potassium and contain proper amounts of different nutrients.

When taking a look at the carb numbers below, remember that a large portion, or about at least 78 percent of the carbs in avocado, are fiber. Hence, they contain little or almost no digestible net carbs. They contain 13 grams of carbs for every cup, or 8.5 grams per 100 grams.

Olives (6%)

The olive is another nutritious and delicious high-fat fruit. It's high in iron and copper and contains a good amount of vitamin E. It contains about two grams of carbs for every ounce, or six grams for every 100 grams.

Strawberries (8%)

Strawberries are among the least carb-heavy and most nutrient-filled fruits you can eat. They're high in vitamin C, manganese, and different cancer prevention agents. They contain about 11 grams of carbs for every cup, or eight grams for every 100 grams.

Grapefruit (11%)

Grapefruits are citrus fruits that are very similar to oranges. They're high in carotene antioxidants and vitamin C. They contain about

There are 13 grams of carbs in half of a grapefruit, or 11 grams for every 100 grams.

Apricots (11%)

The apricot is an extraordinarily tasty fruit. Every apricot contains few carbohydrates, plus a lot of potassium and vitamin. Two apricots contain about two grams of carbs, or there are 11 grams for every 100 grams.

Other Low-Carb Fruits

Lemons

Kiwis

Oranges

Nuts and Seeds

Nuts and seeds are exceptionally prominent on low-carb diets. They will, in general, be low in carbs, yet high in fat, fiber, protein, and different micro vitamins. Nuts are frequently eaten as snacks, while seeds are utilized for adding crunch to recipes and salads. Also, nut and seed flours—for example, coconut flour, almond flour, and flaxseed—are regularly used to make low-carb loaves of bread and other prepared meals.

Almonds (22%)

Almonds are unimaginably delicious and crunchy. They're full of fiber and vitamin E and are one of the world's ideal sources of magnesium, a mineral that the vast majority don't get enough of. Additionally, almonds are fantastically satisfying and have been proven to improve weight loss in some research. They contain six grams of grams for every ounce, or 22 grams for every 100 grams.

Walnuts (14%)

The walnut is another delicious sort of nut. It contains different nutrients and is exceptionally high in alpha-linolenic acid (ALA), a kind of omega-3 fatty acid. Walnuts contain four grams of carbs for every ounce, or 14 grams for every 100 grams.

Peanuts (16%)

Peanuts are, in fact, legumes, yet will, in general, be prepared and consumed the same way as nuts.

They're high in magnesium, fiber, vitamin E, and other essential vitamins and minerals.

Chia Seeds (44%)

Chia seeds are, as of now, among the world's most well-known health foods. They're loaded with numerous essential vitamins and can be utilized in different low-carb-friendly menus.

Also, they're one of the most powerful sources of dietary fiber on the planet.

When taking a look at the carb numbers below, remember that about 86 percent of the carbs in chia seeds are fiber. Hence, they contain few digestible net carbs. They contain about 12 grams of carbs for every ounce, or 44 grams for every 100 grams.

Other Low-Carb Nuts and Seeds

Hazelnuts

Macadamia nuts

Cashews

Coconuts

Pistachios

Flaxseeds

Pumpkin seeds

Sunflower seeds

Dairy

If you're the type of person who tolerates dairy, then full-fat dairy products are great low-carb foods. In any case, make sure to peruse the label and abstain from anything with extra/added sugar.

Cheese (1.3%)

Cheese is a delicious low-carb food and can be eaten both raw and as an ingredient for preparing other meals. Furthermore, it goes exceptionally well with meat, for example, over a bun-less burger.

Cheese is profoundly nutritious. A single thick cut contains a comparative measure of nutrients to a whole glass of milk. It contains 0.4 grams of carbs per cup, or 1.3 grams per 100 grams (cheddar).

Heavy Cream (3%)

Heavy cream contains few carbs and little protein; however, it's high in dairy fat.

A few people on a low-carb diet add it in their coffee or use it in recipes. A bowl of berries with a decent amount of whipped cream can be a sweet low-carb dessert. It contains one gram of carb for every ounce, or three grams for every 100 grams.

Full-Fat Yogurt (5%)

Full-fat yogurt is incredibly healthy, containing a significant number of the same nutrients as whole milk.

On account of its live cultures, yogurt is likewise loaded with helpful probiotic bacteria. It contains 11 grams of carbs for each eight-ounce container, or five grams for every 100 grams.

Greek Yogurt (4%)

Greek yogurt, sometimes called strained yogurt, is highly different from regular yogurt. It's high in numerous helpful nutrients, particularly protein. It contains six grams of carbs for each six-ounce cup, or four grams for every 100 grams.

Fats and Oil

Numerous healthy fats and oils are adequate on a low-carb, genuine food-based diet.

Be that as it may, stay away from refined vegetable oils like corn oil or soybean as these are exceptionally unhealthy when consumed excessively.

- **Margarine/Butter (zero)**

Margarine, which was once demonized for its high saturated fat, has been making a rebound. You should go with grass-fed margarine since it's higher in specific nutrients. It contains zero carbs.

- **Extra Virgin Olive Oil (zero)**

Extra virgin olive oil is one of the most beneficial fats. It's a major ingredient in the heart-healthy Mediterranean diet, stacked with amazing cancer prevention agents and anti-inflammatory compounds. It contains zero carbs.

- **Coconut Oil (zero)**

Coconut oil is an excellent and healthy fat stuffed with medium-chain fatty acids that have powerful, helpful benefits for your digestion. These fatty acids have been proven to diminish hunger, support fat burning, and help individuals lose tummy fat. It contains zero carbs.

Other Examples of Low-Carb-Friendly Fats include:

Tallow

Avocado Oil

Lard

Beverages

Most beverages without sugar are superbly satisfactory on a low-carb diet. Remember that fruit juices are high in sugar and carbs and ought to be avoided.

• Water (zero)

Water ought to be your go-to drink, regardless of whatever the rest of your diet looks like. It contains zero carbs.

• Coffee (zero)

Coffee is healthy and one of the largest sources of dietary antioxidants. Also, coffee consumers have been shown to live more and have a lower risk of some severe ailments, including type 2 diabetes, Parkinson's disease, and Alzheimer's. It contains zero carbs.

• Tea (zero)

Tea, particularly green tea, has been examined thoroughly and proven to have different noteworthy medical advantages. It might even slightly support the burning of fat. It contains zero carbs.

• Club Soda/Carbonated Water (zero)

Club soda is fundamentally water with added carbon dioxide. It's completely satisfactory as long as it has no sugar. Check the label to ensure it is sugar-free. It contains zero carbs.

Herbs and Condiments

There is a great variety of delicious spices, herbs, and condiments. Most of them contain very low carbs but contain powerful nutritional content and help add flavor to your meal. Some of the notable examples include salt, pepper, ginger, mustard, garlic, cinnamon, and oregano.

3.2 Benefits of having a shopping list.

Many times, we think we have a good grasp of grocery shopping such that we can head over to the store with an imaginary store in our heads. However, having a shopping list has its advantages. Beyond saving you time and money, it also makes you shop healthier and smarter. When we go to the store without planning, impulse buying is bound to happen, leading to us sometimes buying some unhealthy food items, or even completely forgetting to buy some of the things we need.

Here are a few reasons why you should have a shopping list:

Saves you time: Whenever we shop for groceries, we often spend money on impulse buying. Rather than filling your cart with all kinds of tempting and flashy items, a shopping list helps you stick with only the needed food items. When you don't fall for the temptation of buying all sorts of things, you will be saving more money.

Helps with meal planning: A shopping list assists in meal planning. When you sit down to write a list, you get to think and plan for what you need for the whole week. Beyond just buying essential food items, you also get to research interesting recipes and come up with new meal ideas. This benefit makes writing a shopping list more interesting and shopping much more fun.

Reduces food waste: Many times, a good portion of the food items that we buy go to waste. This is because often our eyes are bigger than our stomach when we purchase food items like fresh fruits and vegetables.

These food items are highly perishable which means they'll get discarded once they go bad. When you have a shopping list, you can confidently buy the right quantities of food that you can eat without having so much going to waste.

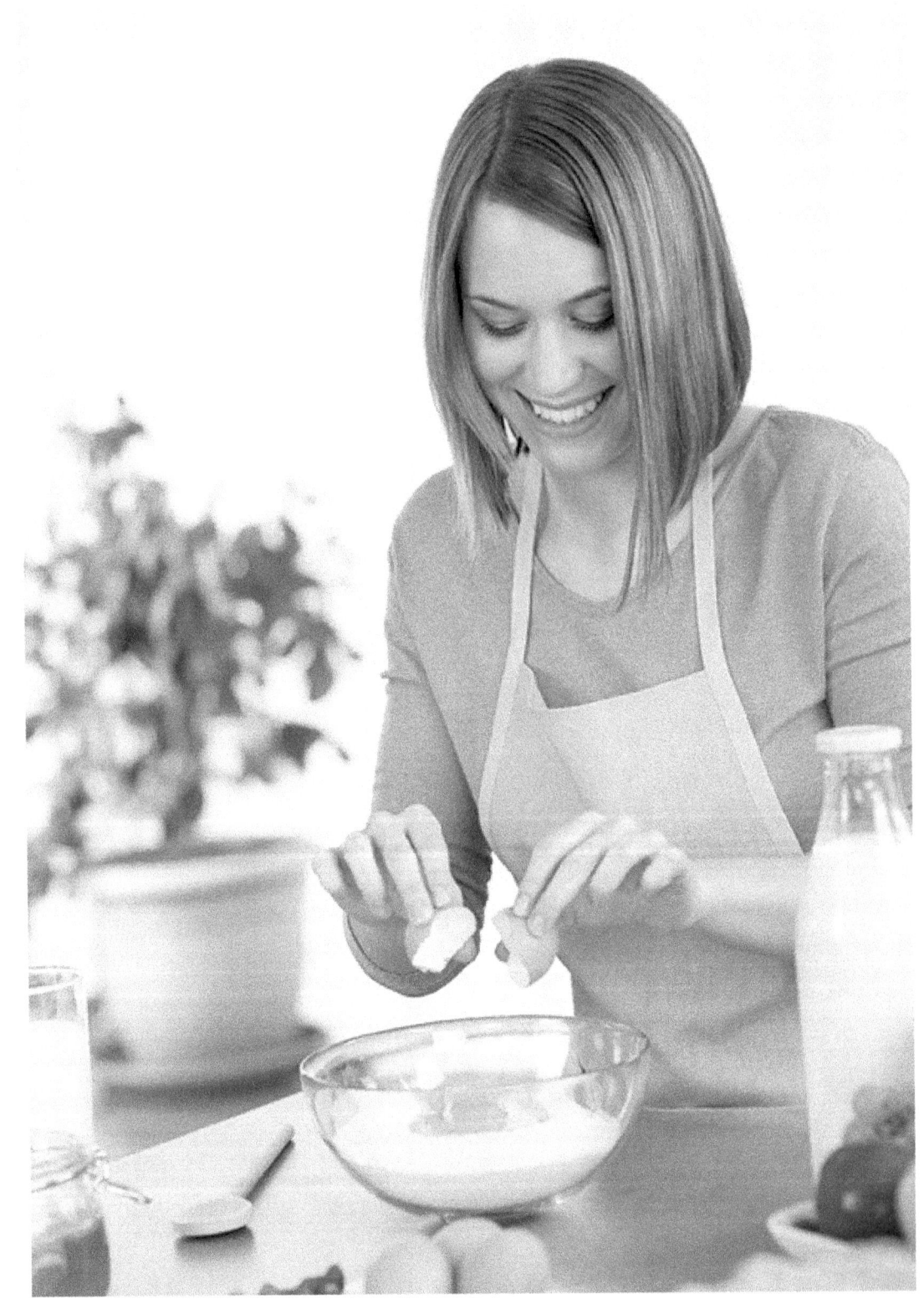

Chapter 4: Simple and Easy Recipes to Start (7-Day Meal Plan)

4.1 This section briefly discusses recipes you can eat while on the keto diet so that beginners will not be overwhelmed. They are recipes that are simple and easy to make that you can eat for a whole week.

4.2

Beyond the fact that these recipes are good for your health. There are other benefits that they bring along. Some of these benefits include:

- Easy to prepare: As opposed to popular thinking that preparing keto diet recipes are difficult to make, keto diet recipes are easy to prepare. All it takes is good planning.
- Flexibility: There's room for experimentation, revisions and customization in preparing these recipes.
- Delicious: These recipes are made using tasty ingredients that will leave you wanting more and more.
- Look good: Keto recipes don't have to look terrible, they are in fact very appealing.
- Not expensive: Going on the keto diet is not expensive. Many of the recipes can be prepared at home thereby saving you extra cash that would have been spent eating out.

4.3

Here's a simple seven-day meal plan for you to follow. Don't forget that the point of the diet is to consume a whole lot of fat, low carbs, and a moderate amount of protein. Ways to prepare some of these recipes are included in later chapters. However, you can use the internet and find out how to cook any of the recipes mentioned here that are not explained in the book.

DAY 1

Breakfast: Cilantro and avocado with scrambled egg lettuce wrap

Snack: Grilled chicken with olive oil dressing with kale salad

Lunch: Chicken-avocado lettuce wraps

Snack: Bell pepper with guacamole

Dinner: Cauliflower rice with steak

DAY 2

Breakfast: Baked egg in an avocado cup

Snack: Cold cut turkey roll-ups or sliced cheese

Lunch: Tuna salad and some green salad

Snack: Macadamia nuts

Dinner: Broccoli or Chinese beef

DAY 3

Breakfast: Full-fat Greek yogurt topped with chia seeds and crushed walnuts

Snack: Turkey jerky (specifically look for the type that has no sugar)

Lunch: Cauliflower fried rice

Snack: Sliced cheese

Dinner: Sautéed mushroom with roast beef and zucchini

DAY 4

Breakfast: Blackberry protein shake with almond butter with kale

Snack: Bacon deviled eggs

Lunch: Chicken tenders made using almond flour on a bed of greens with goat cheese and cucumbers

Snack: Zucchini parmesan chips

Dinner: Grilled shrimp topped with lemon butter sauce and some asparagus

DAY 5

Breakfast: Fried eggs and bacon with a side of greens

Snack: Celery sticks dipped in almond butter

Lunch: Grass-fed burger in a lettuce "bun" with avocado and a side salad

Snack: Half cup of coconut chips

Dinner: Meatloaf served on a bed of watercress salad

DAY 6

Breakfast: Feta cheese and spinach omelet

Snack: Bacon-wrapped asparagus

Lunch: Chicken wings with celery sticks

Snack: Cocoa coconut milk smoothie

Dinner: Bone broth recipe

DAY 7

Breakfast: Full-fat Greek yogurt with pumpkin seeds and coconut chips

Snack: Peanut butter fat bombs

Lunch: Chicken salad wraps

Snack: Cheese crisp

Dinner: Grilled salmon and a side of cauliflower rice

Your Quick-Start Action Step:

Carefully draft out your shopping list of things you'll need to get started on the diet. It doesn't have to be bulky, just ensure it contains enough items to successfully get you started.

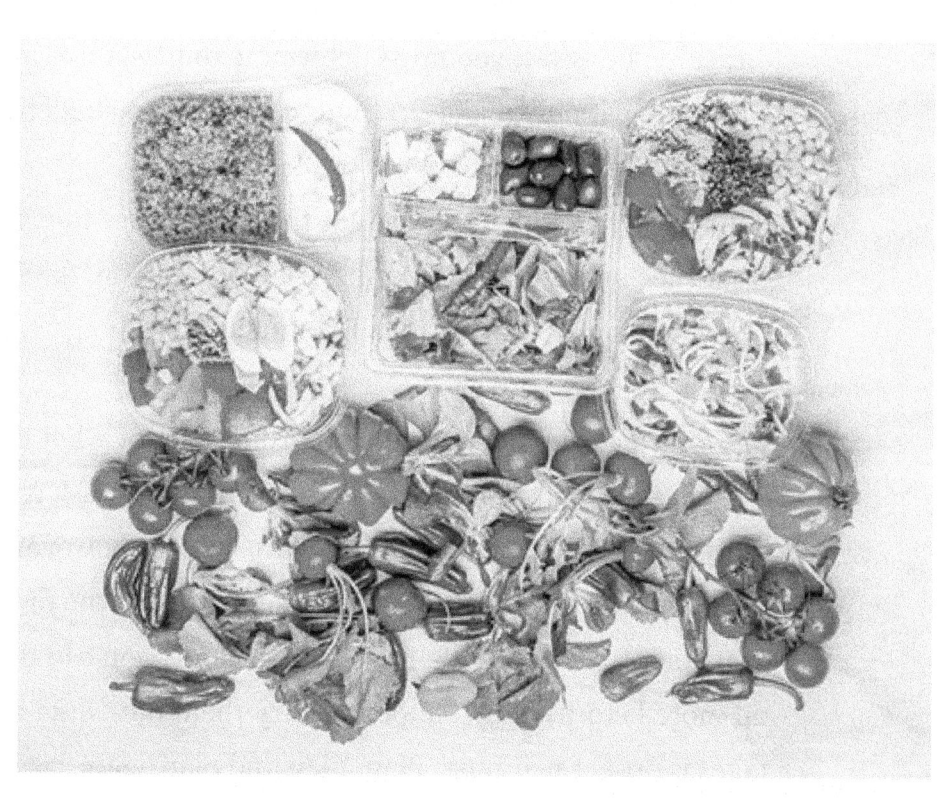

Chapter 5: The Recipes

5.1 The next few chapters are about some of the recipes you can take on the keto diet. These recipes are not just low in carb, they are equally delicious and pleasing to the eye. Going on the keto diet does not equate to eating unappealing meals. Feel free to experiment in your kitchen, just ensure you don't exceed your carb limit.

5.2 When you initially start your diet, it is normal to experience some difficulty; however, you must determine to never give up.
Having to eat only about 20 to 30 carbs can be challenging, especially at the start. Determination is what it takes.
Your body will equally show that there's changes in what you eat, that is what the "keto flu is all about." There'll be many days of weakness and being fatigued, it's all normal. Eventually, your body will adjust to it.

5.3 Your calorie intake is an important part of what determines weight loss or gain, and that is the reason why you must watch it. For many individuals, by just reducing the carb intake, however, if you intend to have a healthy lifestyle you need to keep up with the diet.
You don't have to use the recipes here alone, you can do further research on more keto-friendly recipes and try them out while on your diet. All it takes is proper planning. Plan, plan and plan again.

Your Quick Start Action Step:
Scan through the recipes in the next set of chapters to get a general idea on how to plan into your routine and schedule.

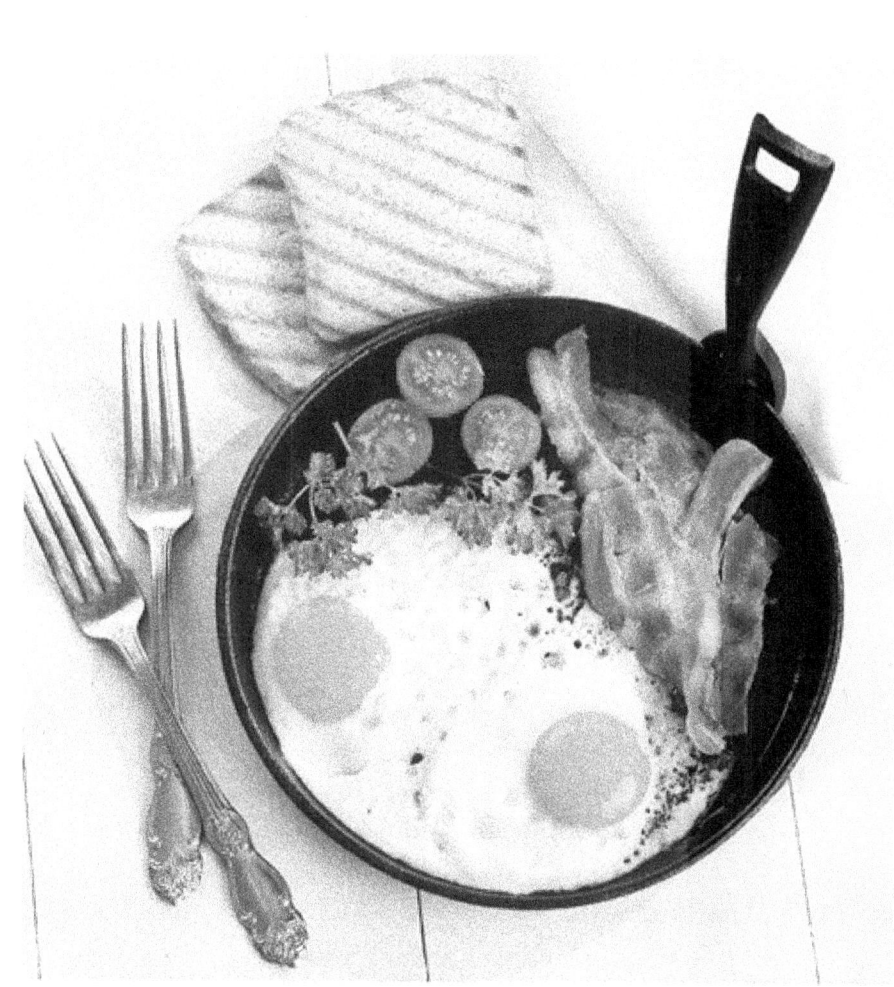

Chapter 6: Breakfast

Keto Frittata With Fresh Spinach

This dish is more than beautiful; it is delicious yet easy to prepare. Spinach, sausage, eggs or bacon, and vegetables all contribute to making this a glorious meal both for the eyes and the tummy. It's a gold star on the keto diet list.

Ingredients

5 oz. diced bacon or chorizo

Eight eggs

Salt and pepper

2 tablespoons butter, for frying

8 oz. fresh spinach

5 oz. shredded cheese

1 cup heavy whipping cream

Instructions

- Preheat the oven until it gets to about 350°F (175°C).
- Then fry the bacon in margarine at medium-high heat until it's crispy. Add the spinach to the bacon and keep stirring until it wilts. Remove the pan from the heat and keep it aside.
- Whisk the eggs and the cream and pour into an oiled baking dish (9×9 inches) or in separate ramekins.
- Add the bacon, cheese, and spinach on top of it and place it right in the middle of the oven.
- Bake for 25 or 30 minutes or till it is set in the middle and golden

brown on top.
- You could try it with shredded red or green cabbage with homemade dressing. Have a delicious breakfast.

Nutritional information:

Net carbs: 2% (4 g)

Fiber: 1 g

Fat: 81% (59 g)

Protein: 16% (27 g)

Kcal: 661

Lemon-Cashew Smoothie

The cashew milk with the heavy cream combines to create a tasty smoothie that is good enough to refresh and still makes for a great breakfast or snack. By adding a few ice cubes, it will be like enjoying a rich citrus sorbet rather than a healthy breakfast. A couple of leaves of fresh mint will also enhance the fresh flavor.

Ingredients

1 cup unsweetened cashew milk

1/4 cup heavy (whipping) cream

1/4 cup freshly squeezed lemon juice

1 scoop plain protein powder

1 tablespoon coconut oil

1 teaspoon sweetener

Instructions

- Put the heavy cream, cashew milk, lemon juice, protein powder, coconut oil, and sweetener in a blender and blend until smooth.
- Pour into a glass and serve immediately.
- Almond milk or coconut milk are also excellent choices instead of cashew milk if you prefer those products. Each type of milk adds a slightly different flavor to the smoothie, so try them all to get the right combination for your palate.

Nutritional information:

Net carbs: 7% (15 g)

Fiber: 4 g

Fat: 80% (45 g)

Protein: 13% (29 g)

Kcal: 503

Nut Medley Granola

Homemade granola is incredibly versatile. It is a treat to have ready-made for breakfast, snacks, and as a healthy topping for a creamy cup of Greek yogurt. The mix and amount of nuts in this recipe create a wonderful keto macro; however, you can add or omit different ingredients as you wish. Don't add dried fruits though, because they are very high in carbs.

Ingredients

2 cups shredded unsweetened coconut

1 cup sliced almonds

1 cup raw sunflower seeds

1/2 cup raw pumpkin seeds

1/2 cup walnuts

1/2 cup melted coconut oil

10 drops liquid stevia

1 teaspoon ground cinnamon

1/2 teaspoon ground nutmeg

Instructions

- Preheat the oven to 250°F. Line two baking sheets with parchment paper and set aside.
- Toss together the almonds, shredded coconut, sunflower seeds, pumpkin seeds, and walnuts in a large bowl until mixed.
- In a small bowl, stir the coconut oil, cinnamon, stevia, and nutmeg until blended.
- Pour the coconut oil mixture and the nut mixture together and blend using your hands until the nuts are well coated.
- Transfer the granola mixture to baking sheets and spread it out evenly.
- Bake the granola. Ensure you stir every 10 to 15 minutes until the mixture turns golden brown and is crunchy.
- Move the granola to a large bowl and allow it to cool, tossing frequently to break up the large pieces. You can store the granola in containers in the refrigerator or freezer for up to one month.

Nutritional information:

Net carbs: 10% (10 g)

Fiber: 6 g

Fat: 80% (38 g)

Protein: 10% (10 g)

Kcal: 391

Bacon-Artichoke Omelet

Omelets are not just for breakfast, and this vegetable- and bacon-packed beauty is hearty enough for a light dinner. If you add a nice mixed green salad to the plate, you won't go over your carbs because the combination with the omelet should still be an excellent keto macro. If you have leftovers, try them cold the next day for a snack or lunch.

Ingredients

6 eggs, beaten

2 tablespoons heavy (whipping) cream

8 bacon slices, cooked and chopped

1 tablespoon olive oil

1/4 cup chopped onion

1/2 cup chopped artichoke hearts (canned, packed in water)

Sea salt

Freshly ground black pepper

Instructions

- In a small bowl, whisk the eggs, bacon and heavy cream until well blended, and set aside.
- Place a large skillet over medium-high heat and add olive oil.
- Sauté the onion until tender, about 3 minutes.
- Pour the egg mixture into the skillet. Swirl it for 1 minute.

- Cook the omelet. Lift the edges using a spatula to let the uncooked egg flow underneath for 2 minutes.
- Sprinkle the artichoke hearts on top and flip the omelet. Cook for 4 minutes more, until the egg is firm. Flip the omelet over again, so the artichoke hearts are on top.
- Remove from the heat, cut the omelet into quarters, and season with salt and black pepper. Transfer the omelet to plates and serve.

Nutritional information:

Net carbs: 5% (5 g)

Fiber: 2 g

Fat: 80% (39 g)

Protein: 15% (17 g)

Kcal: 435

Keto Blt With Cloud Bread

Whenever you say "BLT," the atmosphere begins to change! You can have it alongside the great fluffy cloud bread, popularly called "oopsie bread." It's a grain-free and gluten-free bread. A taste will leave you wanting more!

Ingredients

1 pinch salt

1/2 tablespoon baking powder

4 1/4 oz. cream cheese

1/2 tablespoons ground psyllium husk powder

1/4 cream of tartar (optional)

3 eggs

Toppings

2 oz. lettuce

1 tomato, thinly sliced

8 tablespoons mayonnaise

5 oz. bacon

Fresh basil (optional)

Cloud bread

Instructions

- Preheat the oven until 30°F (15°C).
- Then separate the eggs. Separate the egg whites from the yolks and put them in separate bowls.
- Whip the egg whites together with salt (with cream of tartar, if you want to use any) until they are very stiff. You can do this using a handheld electric mixer. You should be able to turn over the bowl without the egg whites moving.
- Add some cream cheese to the egg yolks and mix. To make the oopsie more bread-like, add some baking powder (optionally, you can also add psyllium seed husk).
- Gently fold all the egg whites into the egg yolk mixture in such a way that there is air in the egg whites.
- Put about 8 oopsie bread pieces on a paper-lined baking tray.
- Bake in the middle of the oven for up to 25 minutes until they look golden.

Building the BLT

- Fry the bacon using a skillet at medium-high heat until it's crispy.
- Turn the oopsie bread piece upside down.
- Spread one or two tablespoons of mayonnaise on each piece.

- Place the lettuce, fried slices of bacon, tomato, and some finely chopped fresh basil in layers in the middle of each bread.

Nutritional information:

Net carbs: 3% (4 g)

Fiber: 1 g

Fat: 88% (48 g)

Protein: 9% (11 g)

Kcal: 498

Peanut Butter Cup Smoothie

If you're a lover of the famous candy featuring chocolate and peanut butter, then you will enjoy the same flavor blend for breakfast or even as a filling snack. If you want a more chocolatey taste, then add a teaspoon of good-quality cocoa powder and a couple of drops of liquid stevia. These additions will not add any fat, protein, or carbs to the smoothie

Ingredients

1 cup water

3/4 cup coconut cream

1 scoop chocolate protein powder

2 tablespoons natural peanut butter

2 ice cubes

Instructions

- Put the coconut cream, water, protein powder, peanut butter, and

ice in a blender and blend until smooth.
- Pour into 2 glasses and serve immediately.

Nutritional Information

Net carbs: 2% (4 g)

Fiber: 5 g

Fat: 70% (40 g)

Protein: 20% (30 g)

Kcal: 486

Keto Mexican Scrambled Eggs

You can spice up your breakfast with this sumptuous keto egg meal. Tomatoes, jalapeños, and scallions can be used to enhance the scrambled eggs with the right quantity of zing; this is a great way to start your day.

Ingredients

1 scallion

6 eggs

Salt and pepper

1 tomato, finely chopped

2 tablespoons butter, for frying

3 oz. shredded cheese

2 pickled jalapeños, finely chopped

Instructions

- Start by chopping the scallions, tomatoes, and jalapeños. Fry them in butter for about 3 minutes on medium heat.
- Break the eggs and pour into a pan. Scramble for about 2 minutes. Add some cheese and seasonings.
- Serve with crisp lettuce, avocado, and dressing to make it more colorful.

Nutritional information:

Net carbs: 3% (2 g)

Fiber: 1 g

Fat: 72% (18 g)

Protein: 24% (14 g)

Kcal: 221

Classic Bacon And Eggs

This is one of the best keto breakfast ever. Enhance your bacon and egg meal with this style. You can eat as many eggs as you need to feel satisfied.

Ingredient

5 oz. bacon, in slices

8 eggs

Fresh parsley (optional)

Cherry tomatoes (optional)

Instruction

- Fry the bacon using a pan at medium-high heat until it is crispy. Remove the fried bacon and set it aside on a plate and leave the rendered fat inside the pan.
- Use the same pan you used in frying the bacon to fry the eggs. Place the pan over medium heat and beat your egg into the bacon fats (alternatively, you can break the eggs into a cup and gently pour into the pan to avoid splattering hot grease).
- Cook the eggs whichever way you like. For eggs cooked over easy, turn the eggs over after some minutes, then cook for one more minute. For sunny-side up, allow the eggs to fry on one side and cover the pan to ensure they get cooked on top.
- You should cut the cherry tomatoes and fry at the same time.
- Add salt and pepper to taste.

Nutritional information:

Net carbs: 2% (1 g)

Fiber: 0 g

Fat: 75% (22 g)

Protein: 23% (15 g)

Kcal: 272

Keto Mushroom Omelet

If you need an easy and quick way to start your day, then this mushroom omelet is for you. It is super healthy and only takes a few minutes to prepare. You can enjoy this meal for breakfast; it also passes for lunch and dinner.

Ingredients

3 mushrooms

3 eggs

Salt and pepper

1 oz. butter, for frying

1/5 yellow onion

1 oz. shredded cheese

Instructions

- Beat the egg into a bowl and mix with pepper and a pinch of salt. Use a fork to whisk the egg until it is smooth and frothy.
- Add some salt and spices.
- Melt some margarine into a frying pan. When it melts, add the egg mixture. By the time the omelet starts to cook and get firm, but still has some raw egg, sprinkle mushrooms, cheese, and onion on top.
- Use a spatula to ease around the edges of the omelet gently and fold it over in equal halves. Once the color begins to change to golden brown beneath, remove the pan from the heat and set the omelet on a plate.
- Serve the omelet alongside a crispy green salad.

Nutritional information:

Net carbs: 3% (4 g)

Fiber: 1 g

Fat: 77% (43 g)

Protein: 20% (25 g)

Kcal: 510

Iced Tea

Cold and refreshing iced tea. It is thirst quenching; hence, you won't notice the absence of sugar. Have the feel of summer all year round with this great beverage.

Ingredient

1 tea bag

1 cup ice cubes

2 cups cold water

Your choice of flavorings, e.g., fresh mint or sliced lemon

Instructions

- Add the tea to half of the cold water and flavoring in a mug and refrigerate for about 1 to 2 hours.
- Remove the tea bag as well as the flavoring. You can replace the flavoring if you want.
- Add the other half of the cold water and serve with plenty of ice cubes.

Nutritional information:

Net carbs: 0% (0 g)

Fiber: 0 g

Fat: 0% (0 g)

Protein: 0% (0 g)

Kcal: 0

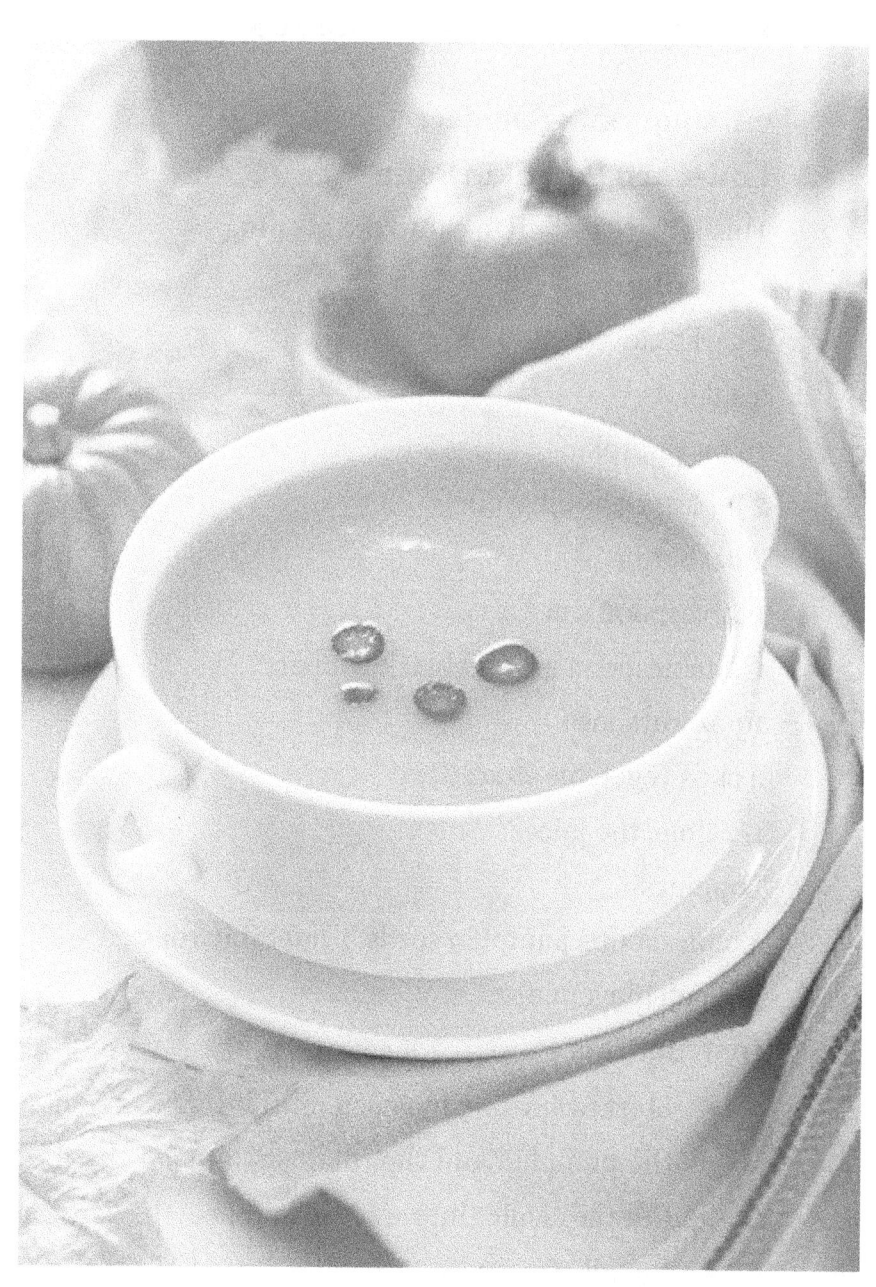

Chapter 7: Soups and Salads

7.1 Soups and Salads

Low-Carb Pumpkin Soup

This is a great soup to eat in the evening.

Ingredients

2 garlic cloves

2 shallots

10 oz. pumpkins

2 tablespoons olive oil

8 oz. butter

1 tablespoon salt

1/2 tablespoon ground black pepper

10 oz. rutabaga

2 cups vegetable stock

1/2 lime, the juice

Toppings

4 tablespoons pumpkin seeds, preferably roasted

3/4 cup mayonnaise

Instructions

- Start by heating the oven until it gets to about 400°F (200°C). Peel the pumpkin and the rutabaga and cut the flesh into small cubes. Cut the shallot into wedges and peel the garlic as well.
- Put all of them into a baking dish. Add some salt, pepper, and olive oil.
- Roast them in the oven for about 25 to 30 minutes. Alternatively, you could also try frying using medium-high heat with a large pan until both the pumpkin and the turnip get soft.
- Put the roasted veggies into a pot. Add vegetable stock or water and leave it to boil. Leave it to simmer for some minutes after which you

- can remove it from the stove.
- Add some butter, divided into cubes. Using a hand blender, mix the soup. Add salt and pepper to taste, juice, and herbs.
- You can have the soup served with mayonnaise, parmesan croutons, or roasted pumpkin seeds.
- Try to make it spicy. Cumin, chili, and some other spices can be used in making this soup. Add some freshly grated ginger a few minutes before serving; it will bring a new kind of twist to the flavor.

Nutritional information:

Net carbs: 6% (14 g)

Fiber: 3 g

Fat: 91% (88 g)

Protein: 3% (6 g)

Kcal: 865

Homemade Chicken Stock

Chicken has a great flavor. You can use it in making stews and sauces. Make a great stew using the chicken stock, and you have a nutrient-filled meal.

Ingredients

1 chicken

1 leek

1 carrot

1 bay leaf

1 yellow onion

1 tablespoon white peppercorn

1/2 cup dry white wine (optional)

2 tablespoons olive oil

2 garlic cloves

Salt

6 cups water

Instructions

- Peel and grate your vegetables into smaller pieces.
- Use olive oil in a big pot to brown the vegetables; you should use an enamel cast pot. Brown them until they have a beautiful color.
- Divide the chicken into equal halves. Pour some spices and water into the pot, cover the pot, reduce the heat, and allow it to simmer for up to 2 hours.
- Remove the chicken and extract the bones until you have just meat left. If you love the chicken skin crispy, then you should spread the chicken skin on an oven sheet lined with clean parchment paper.
- Add some spices to taste, then bake using the oven at about 400°F (200°C) for at least 15 minutes, or better still, until they are crispy.
- Break the chicken bones into smaller pieces and pour back into the pot. Allow it to simmer for 3 more hours.
- Filter your stock using a fine strainer and pour the stock into the pot. Reduce it to about half or more (depending on how rich you want your stock). The stock is not meant to be overcooked; allow it to simmer using medium-low heat. Add some salt towards the end.
- You can have this stored in your refrigerator for 2 to 3 days or freeze it in smaller containers for at least 3 months. It is awesome to use it as a natural flavor enhancer in sauces, pots, and soups.

Nutritional information:

Net carbs: 1% (0.5 g)

Fiber: 0 g

Fat: 81% (13 g)

Protein: 18% (7 g)

Kcal: 145

Blt Salad

The servings of this salad are quite small, but the combination of ingredients packs an intense flavor burst. Using bacon fat in the dressing rather than olive oil adds much more flavor to this already mouthwatering salad. Bacon fat will keep in a sealed container in the refrigerator for up to one week, so save it for other recipes whenever you cook bacon.

Ingredients

2 tablespoons melted bacon fat

2 tablespoons red wine vinegar

Freshly ground black pepper

4 cups shredded lettuce

1 tomato, chopped

6 bacon slices, cooked and chopped

2 hardboiled eggs, chopped

1 tablespoon roasted unsalted sunflower seeds

1 teaspoon toasted sesame seeds

1 cooked chicken breast, sliced (optional)

Instructions

- Use a medium bowl to whisk the vinegar and bacon fat until emulsified. Season with black pepper.
- Add the tomato and lettuce to the bowl and toss the vegetables with the dressing.
- Divide the salad into 4 plates and top each with equal amounts of egg, bacon, sesame seeds, sunflower seeds, and chicken (if using). Serve.

Nutritional information:

Net carbs: 7% (4 g)

Fiber: 2 g

Fat: 76% (18 g)

Protein: 17% (1 g)

Kcal: 228

Cauliflower-Cheddar Soup

Cauliflower is a popular vegetable that can be eaten on the keto diet in many recipes, like this creamy soup. Cauliflower is a good source of manganese, vitamins C and K, and omega-3 fatty acids which improve brain function, help support digestion, and promote a healthy heart. You should choose a snow- white head of cauliflower with crisp green leaves and no brown spots.

Ingredients

1/2 sweet onion, chopped

1 cup heavy (whipping) cream

1 head cauliflower, chopped

1/4 cup butter

4 cups herbed chicken stock

1/2 teaspoon ground nutmeg

Sea salt

Freshly ground black pepper

1 cup shredded cheddar cheese

Instructions

- Place a large pot over medium heat and add butter.
- Sauté the onion and cauliflower until tender and lightly browned, about 10 minutes.
- Add the nutmeg and chicken stock to the pot and bring the liquid to a boil.
- Then reduce the heat and allow it to simmer until the vegetables are soft.
- Remove the pot from the heat and stir in the heavy cream. Purée the soup with a food processor or an immersion blender until smooth.
- Salt and pepper the soup. Serve topped with the cheddar cheese.

Nutritional information:

Net carbs: 9% (4 g)

Fiber: 2 g

Fat: 81% (21 g)

Protein: 12% (8 g)

Kcal: 227

Wild Mushroom Soup

The warm mushroom keto soup is a delight. It is particularly creamy and smooth.

Ingredients

5 oz. portabella mushrooms

5 oz. shiitake mushrooms

5 oz. oyster mushrooms

4 oz. butter

1 garlic clove

1 cup heavy whipping cream

1 tablespoon white wine vinegar

3 cups water

1/2 cup thyme

1/2 lb. celery root

1 vegetable bouillon cube or chicken bouillon cube

Fresh parsley (optional)

Instructions

- Wash, trim, and cut the mushrooms and celery root. Peel the onion and garlic and finely chop them.
- Sauté the chopped vegetables in margarine using medium heat in a heavy-bottomed saucepan until it turns brown. Reserve some mushroom for serving.
- Add vinegar, thyme, bouillon cube, and water and allow it to boil. Reduce the heat and allow to simmer for up to 15 minutes or until the celery is soft enough.
- Add some cream and puree using an immersion blender until you achieve the fineness you want. Serve it with some pieces of sautéed

- mushroom and finely chopped parsley.
- Feel free to try out some other mushroom types like porcini, chanterelles, and white-buttoned mushrooms.

Nutritional information:

Net carbs: 10% (11 g)

Fiber: 3 g

Fat: 85% (45 g)

Protein: 5% (6 g)

Kcal: 468

Green Gazpacho

This is a great chilled keto soup that you can try during hot summer months. It's simply a blend of all the ingredients into a drinkable soup.

Ingredients

1/2 cup diced celery stalks

1/2 cup presoaked drained cashew nuts

1/2 cup peeled, seeded and sliced cucumber

1/2 cup watercress leaves

5 oz. Romaine lettuce (5 large crisp leaves)

1 garlic clove

1/4 cup extra virgin oil

1 cup chicken broth

1 tablespoon fine salt

Instruction

- Put all ingredients into a blender and keep blending until smooth and creamy. You can serve and enjoy.
- You can soak the cashews in salty water for about 3 hours to minimize the phytic acid content in them, thereby aiding the digestion.

Nutritional information:

Net carbs: 11% (9 g)

Fiber: 2 g

Fat: 82% (29 g)

Protein: 6% (5 g)

Kcal: 311

Spicy Almond And Seed Mix

The spicy almond and seed mix with a blend of cumin are awesome as a snack or even as topping for soups and salads. It is guaranteed to be completely free of additives.

Ingredients

1 cup almonds

2 tablespoons olive oil or coconut oil

1/3 cup sunflower seeds

1/3 cup pumpkin seeds

1 tablespoon ground and crushed fennel or cumin seeds

1/2 tablespoon salt

1 tablespoon chili paste

Instructions

- Preheat the oil in a large frying pan, then add the chili.
- Add the almonds and seeds, then stir thoroughly.
- Sauté for some minutes and add salt. You must note that almonds and seeds are sensitive to heat, so ensure the oil is hot enough to allow the spice flavors to develop. However, ensure the almonds and seeds don't get burnt.
- Allow to cool, then store in a glass container.
- You can serve it as a snack or as a topping with cauliflower soup or as a crispy flavor enhancer.

Nutritional information:

Net carbs: 6% (2 g)

Fiber: 3 g

Fat: 81% (15 g)

Protein: 13% (6 g)

Kcal: 166

Greek Egg And Lemon Soup With Chicken

If you want something creamy without using real cream, try out this Greek recipe, "avgolemono." It is very easy to prepare. All you need is chicken, eggs, cauliflower, and butter.

Ingredients

2 chicken bouillon cubes

1 lb. boneless chicken thighs

1 bay leaf

4 cups water

3/4 lb. cauliflower

4 eggs

1/3 lb. butter

2 tablespoons fresh thyme or fresh parsley

1 lemon—zest and juice

Salt and ground black pepper

Instructions

- Slice the chicken thigh into thin pieces, place it in a saucepan, add some cold water, and boil. Add bay leaf and some bouillon cubes.
- Reduce the heat to medium and allow it to simmer for about 10 minutes or until the chicken is thoroughly cooked.
- Remove the bay leaf and meat from the heat and don't allow the broth to get cold.
- Grate the cauliflower until it resembles rice and put it in the saucepan.
- Increase the heat, add some butter, and boil for a few minutes. Break the eggs into a bowl and add lemon juice.
- Add salt and pepper to taste.
- Reduce the heat and then add the eggs. Stir continuously and allow

to simmer for a few minutes until the soup becomes slightly thick, but don't boil; it will likely curdle.

- Add the chicken back to the soup. Serve with lemon zest and some finely chopped thyme or parsley.

    You can reheat the soup using medium heat until it simmers. But be careful so it doesn't boil. It will still be delicious, but you sure don't want the curdled look.

    Alternatively, you can skip steps 1 and 2 and warm up the poultry in the broth in step 6.

Nutritional information:

Net carbs: 3% (5 g)

Fiber: 2 g

Fat: 79% (54 g)

Protein: 17% (27 g)

Kcal: 620

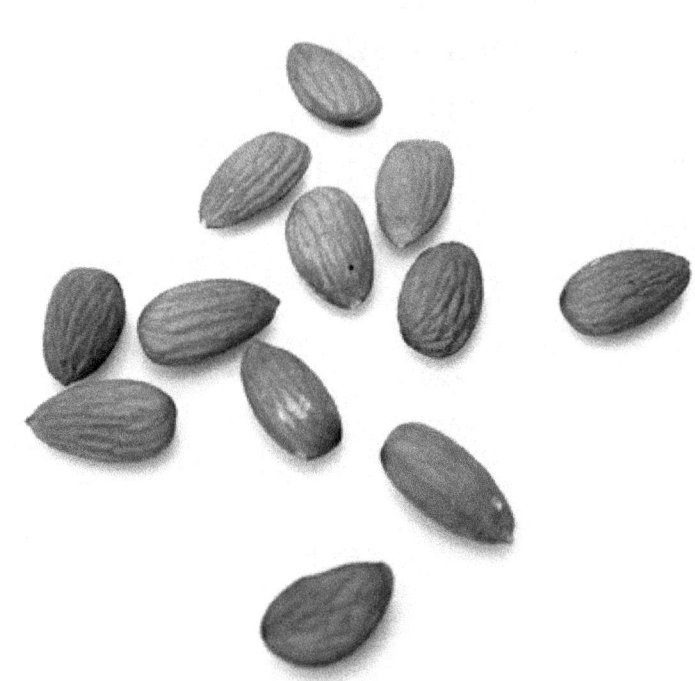

Chapter 8: Snacks and Side Dishes

Low-Carb Cauliflower Rice

If you're missing rice, then here is the perfect low-carb substitute. Cauliflower rice is awesome eaten with Asian dishes and is a good replacement for pasta or couscous. It's neutral and finely textured.

Ingredients

3 oz. butter or coconut oil

25 oz. cauliflower

1/2 tablespoon salt

1/2 tablespoon turmeric (optional)

Instructions

- Use a grater to shred the cauliflower head.
- Melt margarine or coconut oil in a skillet. Add the cauliflower and cook using medium heat for about 5 to 10 minutes or until the riced cauliflower softens.
- Salt it, and optionally, add some turmeric while frying.
- You can cook the grated cauliflower using the microwave. Place it in a glass plate and cover it with a plastic wrap. Microwave it for about 5 to 6 minutes. Mix the butter or coconut oil and allow it to melt.
- You can make your cauliflower rice "au naturel"—skip the turmeric. Or you can use a different herb to spice it up like curry, herb salt, or paprika powder.

Nutritional information:

Net carbs: 11% (6 g)

Fiber: 4 g

Fat: 82% (19 g)

Protein: 7% (4 g)

Kcal: 208

Creamed Green Cabbage

It's soft and easy. It also goes with everything. This creamy keto dish is so good, you'll be tempted to make a whole lot for you to enjoy all week.

Ingredients

25 oz. green cabbage

2 oz. butter

1/2 cup fresh, finely chopped parsley

1 1/4 cups whipping heavy cream

1/2 zest lemon

Salt and pepper

Instructions

- You should start by shredding the cabbage by slicing thinly with a sharp knife or with a food processor.
- Melt the margarine in a frying pan on medium-high heat. Add cabbage and sauté for some minutes until it gets soft and the color changes to golden around the edges.
- Add plenty of whipping cream and allow the cabbage simmer until the cream reduces. Reduce the heat towards the end.

- Add pepper and salt to taste.
- Add some parsley and lemon zest just before serving. If you want to reduce your daily dairy consumption, you can switch the heavy whipping cream with coconut cream or coconut oil.

Nutritional information:

Net carbs: 9% (9 g)

Fiber: 5 g

Fat: 87% (38 g)

Protein: 5% (5 g)

Kcal: 401

Crab Salad-Stuffed Avocado

Depending on the size of your avocados, this decadent dish could be a filling snack or a light lunch. It's perfectly acceptable to use frozen crab if fresh is not available, but be careful to look for real crab meat rather than cheaper imitation products. If using frozen crab, thaw it completely and squeeze out any extra liquid so that your salad isn't soggy.

Ingredients

1 avocado, peeled, halved lengthwise, and pitted

1/2 teaspoon freshly squeezed lemon juice

4 1/2 ounces Dungeness crabmeat

1/2 cup cream cheese

1/4 cup chopped red bell pepper

1/4 cup chopped, peeled English cucumber

1/2 scallion, chopped

1 teaspoon chopped cilantro

Pinch sea salt

Freshly ground black pepper

Instructions

- Brush the cut edges of the avocado with the lemon juice and set the halves aside on a plate.
- In a medium bowl, stir the crabmeat, cream cheese, red pepper, cucumber, scallion, cilantro, salt, and pepper until well mixed.
- Split the crab mixture between the avocado halves and store them, covered with plastic wrap, in the refrigerator until you're ready to serve them (up to 2 days).

Nutritional information:

Net carbs: 10% (10 g)

Fiber: 5 g

Fat: 70% (31 g)

Protein: 20% (19 g)

Kcal: 389

Turkey Rissoles

Chicken is often the first choice for poultry in most home kitchens, but turkey is fabulous tasting, inexpensive, and very healthy. Turkey is low in fat and high in protein. Make sure some of your other recipe ingredients are high in fat so your keto macro is perfect. Turkey can help boost your immunity because it contains an amino acid called tryptophan, which supports the immune system.

Ingredients

1-pound ground turkey

1 scallion, green and white parts, finely chopped

1 teaspoon minced garlic

Pinch sea salt

Pinch freshly ground black pepper

1 cup ground almonds

2 tablespoons olive oil

Instructions

- Preheat the oven to 350°F (175°C). Line a baking sheet with aluminum foil and set it aside.
- In a medium bowl, mix the turkey, scallion, garlic, salt, and pepper until well combined.
- Mold the turkey mixture into 8 patties and flatten them out.
- Place the ground almonds in a shallow bowl and dredge the turkey patties in the ground almonds to coat.
- Place a large skillet over medium heat and add the olive oil.
- Brown the turkey patties on both sides, about 10 minutes in total.
- Transfer the patties to the baking sheet. Bake them until cooked through, flipping them once, about 15 minutes in total.
- Make the whole recipe from start to finish and place the cooled turkey patties in sealed plastic bags and store them in the refrigerator for up to 3 days or the freezer for up to 1 month.
- Take them out of the freezer and thaw for a quick dinner or snack or reheat them right from the refrigerator.

Nutritional information:

Net carbs: 10% (10 g)

Fiber: 5 g

Fat: 70% (31 g)

Protein: 20% (19 g)

Kcal: 389

Roasted Pork Loin With Grainy Mustard Sauce

This is a delicious sauce; you might have to double the amount you make because eating it by the spoonful as a snack is a real treat. It is also stellar with barbecued beef tenderloin or a perfectly roasted lamb rack.

Ingredients

3 tablespoons grainy mustard, such as Pommery

1 (2-pound) boneless pork loin roast

Freshly ground black pepper

3 tablespoons olive oil

Sea salt

1 1/2 cups heavy (whipping) cream

Instructions

- Preheat the oven to 375°F (175°C).
- Season the pork roast all over with sea salt and pepper.
- Place a large skillet over medium-high heat and add the olive oil.
- Roast until all sides turn brown in the skillet. This will take about 6

minutes in total, then place the roast in a baking dish.
- Roast until a meat thermometer put in the thickest part of the roast reads 155°F (72°C), about 1 hour.
- When there are about 15 minutes of roasting time left, place a small saucepan over medium heat and add the heavy cream and mustard.
- Stir the sauce until it simmers, then reduce the heat to low. Simmer the sauce until it is very rich and thick, about 5 minutes.
- Remove the pan from the heat and set aside. Let the pork cool for 10 minutes before you slice and serve with the sauce.

Nutritional information:

Net carbs: 5% (2 g)

Fiber: 0 g

Fat: 70% (29 g)

Protein: 25% (25 g)

Kcal: 368

Portobella Mushroom Pizza

Mozzarella is prepared using a method that spins the milk from the cheese and then cuts it. The method is called pasta filata.

Mozzarella is a great choice for the keto diet. It is high in fat (65 percent), contains about 32 percent protein, and has only three percent carbs.

Ingredients

4 large Portobella mushrooms, stems removed

1/4 cup olive oil

1 teaspoon minced garlic

1 medium tomato, cut into 4 slices

2 teaspoons chopped fresh basil

1 cup shredded mozzarella cheese

Instructions

- Start by preheating the oven to broil. Line a baking sheet with clean aluminum foil and set it aside.
- Using a small bowl, toss the mushroom caps with the olive oil until well coated.
- Use your fingertips to rub the oil in. Avoid breaking the mushrooms.
- Place the mushrooms on the baking sheet, gill-side down, and broil the mushrooms until they are tender on the tops, about 2 minutes.
- Turn the mushrooms over and broil 1 minute more.
- Take out the baking sheet and spread the garlic over each mushroom, top each with a tomato slice, sprinkle with the basil, and also top with the cheese.
Broil the mushrooms till the cheese is melted and bubbly, about 1 minute, and serve.

These pizzas pack a lot of flavors, so you'll need an assertive main course to share the plate with them. Some wonderful options could include Bacon-Wrapped Beef Tenderloin or Sirloin with Blue Cheese Compound Butter. These juicy mushrooms make a tempting snack, as well.

Nutritional information:

Net carbs: 10% (7 g)

Fiber: 3 g

Fat: 71% (20 g)

Protein: 19% (14 g)

Kcal: 251

Low-Carb Eggplant Hash With Eggs

Are you missing the old potato hash? If so, then you should try this one out! A delicious and easy to make keto-friendly meal that the entire household should love.

Ingredients

4 eggs

2 eggplants

2 tablespoons olive oil

1 yellow onion

2 tablespoons butter

8 oz. halloumi cheese or any other cheese that can be fried

1/2 tablespoon Worcestershire sauce (optional)

Instructions

- Peel and finely chop the onion.
- Dice the halloumi cheese and eggplant into 1/2-inch cubes.
  Fry the onion in oil using medium heat until it gets soft. Add eggplant and halloumi and fry until it all turns golden brown.
- Add salt and pepper to taste.
- Fry the eggs using whatever style you wish in another pan. You can optionally serve with some drops Worcestershire sauce.

You should buy small or medium-sized eggplants; they are usually better than the larger ones in terms of flavor.

Nutritional information:

Net carbs: 11% (11 g)

Fiber: 8 g

Fat: 69% (31 g)

Protein: 20% (20 g)

Kcal: 423

Low-Carb Onion Rings

This is one of the easiest recipes you can make. It's simply onion made into rings. They can be eaten alongside chicken, burgers, or anything grilled. It's so simple, yet so delicious.

Ingredients

1 jumbo onion

1 cup almond flour

1 egg

1 tablespoon olive oil

1 tablespoon garlic powder

½ cup grated parmesan cheese

½ tablespoon powder or paprika powder

1 pinch of salt

Instructions

- Start by preheating the oven until it reaches about 400°F (200C).
- Peel and slice the onion into rings that are about 1/5 inch thick.
- Mix all ingredients in a bowl while you beat and whisk the egg in a separate bowl.
- Dip the onion rings into the egg batter and dip in a flour mix as well, one at a time.
- You can put the rings of onions in a baking sheet covered with parchment paper.
- Spray oil on the rings and bake using an oven for about 15 to 20 minutes. If you're using the broiler, ensure you monitor them closely; they're ready once the color changes to golden brown and they are crisp.

Nutritional information:

Net carbs: 7% (5 g)

Fiber: 1 g

Fat: 74% (26 g)

Protein: 19% (15 g)

Kcal: 323

Spicy Keto Roasted Nuts

They're spicy, crunchy, salty, and snacky. These nuts will have your guests asking for more.

Ingredients

8 oz. almonds, walnuts, or pecans.

1 tablespoon coconut oil or olive oil

1 tablespoon chili powder or paprika powder

1 tablespoon ground cumin

1 tablespoon salt

Instructions

- Add all ingredients in a medium frying pan and mix thoroughly. Cook using medium heat until the almonds have been warmed.
- Allow it to cool. Serve as a snack, or eat alongside a drink.
- Store at room temperature in a container with a lid.
  You don't necessarily have to use almonds; you can use other types of nuts, e.g., pecans.

Nutritional information:

Net carbs: 3% (2 g)

Fiber: 4 g

Fat: 92% (29 g)

Protein: 5% (4 g)

Kcal: 281

Keto Cheese Puffs

They're simple, crunchy, and crispy.

Ingredients

5 1/3 oz. Brie cheese (preferably President Brie)

Instructions

- Cut the rind off the Brie cheese and cut it into small 1/2-inch cubes. Ensure you remove the white edge.
- Put some pieces of the brie cheese on a paper. Put on a plate and use a microwave oven to bake at full power for 1 to 2 minutes. You should observe it to ensure it doesn't get burnt. Don't make too many at a time.
- Allow to cool before serving. You can season it with whatever spices you want.

Nutritional information:

Net carbs: 1% (0.2 g)

Fiber: 0 g

Fat: 75% (14 g)

Protein: 25% (10 g)

Kcal: 167

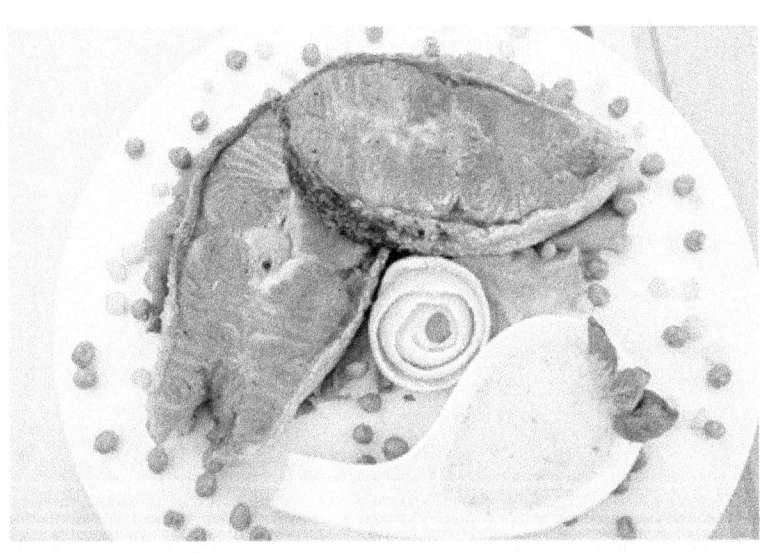

Chapter 9: Fish and Poultry

Keto Salmon With Pesto And Spinach

If you love both salmon and pesto, then this dish is for you.

Ingredients

1 tablespoon green or red pesto

25 oz. salmon

2 oz. grated parmesan cheese

1/6 oz. butter or olive oil

1 lb. fresh spinach

Instructions

- Start by heating the oven until it reaches about 400°F (2000c).
- Grease the baking dish with oil or about half of the butter.
- Add salt and pepper to the salmon fillets and put them in the prepared baking dish, skin-side down.
- Mix the pesto, mayonnaise, and parmesan cheese and spread on top of the salmon.
- Bake the mixture for about 15 to 20 minutes, or until the salmon easily flakes with a fork.
  Meanwhile, you should use the remaining oil or butter to sauté the spinach until it wilts. After 2 minutes, season with pepper and salt.
- You can serve along with the salmon that was baked in the oven.

Nutritional information:

Net carbs: 1% (3 g)

Fiber: 3 g

Fat: 79% (78 g)

Protein: 20% (45 g)

Kcal: 902

Keto Tuna Casserole

You can use this as a good replacement for noodles. It's made with peppers, onions, celery, and can be prepared in about 30 minutes.

Ingredients

1 green bell pepper

2 oz. butter

5 1/3 oz. celery stalks

1 cup mayonnaise

4 oz. freshly shredded parmesan cheese

16 oz. tuna in drained olive oil

1 yellow onion

1 tablespoon chili flakes

Instructions

- Start by preheating the oven until it reaches 400°F (200°C). Finely chop the celery bell, pepper, and onion.
- Fry the chopped ingredients in margarine until it is relatively soft. Add salt and pepper to taste.
- Mix the chili flakes, mayonnaise, parmesan cheese, and tuna in an oiled baking dish. Add some fried vegetables and stir.

- Allow to bake in the oven for about 15 to 20 minutes or until golden brown.

Nutritional information:

Net carbs: 2% (5 g)

Fiber: 3 g

Fat: 80% (83 g)

Protein: 18% (43 g)

Kcal: 953

Keto Baked Salmon With Butter And Lemon

Simply a great meal

Ingredients

2 lbs. salmon

1 tablespoon olive oil

Black ground pepper

1 lemon

7 oz. butter

Instructions

- Start by preheating the oven until it reaches 400°F (200°C).
- Put a little amount of olive oil in the large baking dish. Put the salmon in skin- side down. Add pepper and salt according to your taste.
- Slice the lemon into thin pieces and put it on top of the salmon. Use

- half of the butter to cover the salmon
- Place it on the middle rack of the oven and bake for at least 20 to 30 minutes, or until the salmon looks opaque and easily flakes with a fork.
- Put the remaining butter in a small saucepan and heat until it begins to bubble.
- Remove from the stove and allow to cool for a little while. Gently add some of the lemon juice.
- You can serve the fish with any side dish you want with the lemon butter.

You can try adding lemon zest to your butter.

Nutritional information:

Net carbs: 0% (1 g)

Fiber: 0 g

Fat: 78% (49 g)

Protein: 22% (31 g)

Kcal: 573

Sweet And Sticky Chicken Wings

They have layers of aromas, textures, and flavors that will excite your senses. Crispy and juicy, savory and sweet at the same time. It brings back childhood memories of sticky fingers.

Ingredients

2 lbs. chicken wings

3/4 cup coconut aminos

1 1/2 tablespoon sea salt

1/4 tablespoon onion powder

1/4 tablespoon ground ginger

1/4 tablespoon garlic powder

1/4 tablespoon chili flakes

Instructions

- Start by preheating the oven until it reaches 450°F (230°C).
- Place the chicken wings on a rimmed baking sheet that has wire racks, thicker skin side facing up. The wire racks help enhance the cooking.
- Sprinkle some fine pink Himalayan sea salt or any other salt on the wings.
- Allow the wings to bake for about 45 minutes.
- Using medium heat, heat a medium-sized or large skillet and then add the coconut aminos.
- You can now add the onion powder, garlic powder ginger powder, and some red pepper flakes if you want. Once the sauce begins to simmer, start stirring. Continue occasionally stirring while adjusting the heat accordingly to ensure a gentle simmer.
- Once you notice that the sauce has started thickening (when you stir it, it usually should take only a few seconds to rise and fill your spatula or spoon), you can reduce the heat while the wings finish cooking.
- Put the wings in a large heat-resistant bowl and pour the sauce on them. Serve after you have stirred to coat evenly.

Nutritional information:

Net carbs: 3% (10 g)

Fiber: 3 g

Fat: 5% (3 g)

Protein: 8% (4 g)

Kcal: 67

Keto Chicken And Cabbage Plate

This is an example of a keto dinner that is not complicated.

Ingredients

7 oz. fresh green cabbage

1 lb. rotisserie chicken

1/2 red onion

1/2 cup mayonnaise

1 tablespoon olive oil

Salt and pepper

Instructions

- Cut the cabbage with a sharp knife and place on a plate.
- Slice the onion into thin pieces and put it with the chicken on the same plate. Also add a good quantity of mayonnaise.
- Sprinkle some olive oil on the cabbage.
- Add some pepper and salt to taste.
  You can make use of leftover chicken rather than rotisserie chicken.

Nutritional information:

Net carbs: 3% (7 g)

Fiber: 3 g

Fat: 79% (91 g)

Protein: 19% (48 g)

Kcal: 1041

Simple Fish Curry

Curry is a sauce-based recipe originating in India and adopted by many cultures.

The ubiquitous spice mixture often contains a multitude of ingredients such as cumin, coriander, turmeric, ginger, cloves, paprika, and cinnamon. It's adapted so well to many cuisines because no matter the ingredients used—vegetables, meats, fish, eggs, butter, or coconut—the spices bring the dish together beautifully.

Ingredients

2 tablespoons coconut oil

1 1/2 tablespoons grated fresh ginger

2 teaspoons minced garlic

1 tablespoon curry powder

1/2 teaspoon ground cumin

2 cups coconut milk

16 ounces firm white fish, cut into 1-inch chunks

1 cup shredded kale

2 tablespoons chopped cilantro

Instructions

- Place a large saucepan over medium heat and melt the coconut oil.
- Sauté the ginger and garlic until lightly browned, about 2 minutes.
- Stir the curry powder and cumin and sauté until very fragrant, about 2 minutes.
- Stir in the coconut milk and bring the liquid to a boil.
- Reduce the heat and allow it to simmer for about 5 minutes to infuse the milk with the spices.
- Add the fish and cook until the fish is cooked through about 10 minutes.
- Stir in the kale and cilantro and simmer until wilted, about 2 minutes, and serve.

Nutritional information:

Net carbs: 6% (5 g)

Fiber: 1 g

Fat: 70% (31 g)

Protein: 24% (26 g)

Kcal: 416

Pan-Seared Halibut With Citrus Butter Sauce

Citrus fruits are delicious and are bursting with nutrients. Both lemons and oranges are excellent sources of vitamin C, which boosts the immune system and can help detoxify your body. The acid from citrus is a wonderful addition to most fish and seafood recipes.

Ingredients

4 (5-ounce) halibut fillets, each about 1-inch thick

Sea salt

Freshly ground black pepper

1/4 cup butter

2 teaspoons minced garlic

1 shallot, minced

3 tablespoons dry white wine

1 tablespoon freshly squeezed lemon juice

1 tablespoon freshly squeezed orange juice

2 teaspoons chopped fresh parsley

2 tablespoons olive oil

Instructions

- Dry the fish by patting with paper towels and then lightly season the fillets with salt and pepper. Set aside on a paper towel-lined plate.
- Place a small saucepan over medium heat and melt the butter.
- Sauté the garlic and shallot until tender, about 3 minutes.
- Whisk in the white wine, lemon juice, and orange juice and bring the sauce to a simmer. Cook until it thickens slightly, about 2 minutes.
- Remove the sauce from the heat and stir in the parsley; set aside.
- Place a large skillet over medium-high heat and add olive oil.
- Panfry the fish until lightly browned and just cooked through, turning over once, about 10 minutes in total.
- Serve the fish immediately with a spoonful of sauce for each.

Any firm white-fleshed fish will be delicious with this creamy sauce. Try haddock, tilapia, or sea bass.

Nutritional information:

Net carbs: 1% (2 g)

Fiber: 0 g

Fat: 70% (26 g)

Protein: 29% (22 g)

Kcal: 319

Roasted Salmon With Avocado Salsa

Simple, fresh salsa is often the best topping for a juicy piece of fish, and creamy avocados are a perfect choice for the base. Take the salsa ingredients out of the refrigerator an hour or so before serving the fish, so they come to room temperature.

The taste of the avocado will be much stronger than when this fruit is completely chilled. You can also grill the salmon for this recipe—this fish holds up well under higher heat and does not dry out.

Ingredients for the Salsa

1 avocado, peeled, pitted, and diced

1 scallion, white and green parts, chopped

1/2 cup halved cherry tomatoes

Juice of 1 lemon

Zest of 1 lemon

Ingredients for the Fish

1 teaspoon ground cumin

1/2 teaspoon ground coriander

1/2 teaspoon onion powder

1/4 teaspoon sea salt

Pinch freshly ground black pepper

Pinch cayenne pepper

4 (4-ounce) boneless, skinless salmon fillets

2 tablespoons olive oil

Instructions on how to make the Salsa

- In a small bowl, stir the avocado, scallion, tomatoes, lemon juice, and lemon zest until mixed and set aside.

Instructions on how to bake the Fish

- Preheat the oven to about 400°F (200°C). Line a baking sheet with clean aluminum foil and set aside.
- In a small bowl, stir the cumin, coriander, onion powder, salt, black pepper, and cayenne until well mixed.
- Rub the spice mix on the salmon fillets and place them on the baking sheet.
- Drizzle the fillets with the olive oil and roast the fish until just cooked through, about 15 minutes.
- Serve the salmon alongside the avocado salsa.

Nutritional information:

Net carbs: 5% (4 g)

Fiber: 3 g

Fat: 69% (26 g)

Protein: 26% (22 g)

Kcal: 320

Sole Asiago

Sole is a flatfish, which means both of its eyes are on one side of its head. It looks rather strange, but when filleted, it is delicious. Sole is not a threatened species, but it is overfished in some areas, so it is not as plentiful as it was in the past. This tender, delicate fish freezes very well; if you cannot find fresh fillets, frozen fillets will work, too.

Ingredients

4 (4-ounce) sole fillets

3/4 cup ground almonds

1/4 cup Asiago cheese

2 eggs, beaten

2 1/2 tablespoons melted coconut oil

Instructions

- Preheat the oven to 350°F (175°C). Line a baking sheet with clean parchment paper and set aside.
- Pat the fish dry with paper towels.
- Stir together the ground almonds and cheese in a small bowl.
- Place the bowl with the beaten eggs next to the almond mixture.
- Dredge a sole fillet in the beaten egg and then press the fish into

the almond mixture, so it is completely coated. Place on the baking sheet and repeat until all the fillets are breaded
- Brush both sides of each piece of fish with the coconut oil.
- Bake the sole until it is cooked through, about 8 minutes in total.
- Serve immediately.

Nutritional information:

Net carbs: 5% (6 g)

Fiber: 3 g

Fat: 65% (31 g)

Protein: 30% (29 g)

Kcal: 406

Keto Fajita Chicken Casserole

It's made with great flavors. Perfect for weekends.

Ingredients

7 oz. cream cheese

1 rotisserie chicken

1/3 cup mayonnaise

1 yellow onion

1 red bell pepper

7 oz. shredded pepper

2 tablespoons Tex-Mex seasoning

Salt and pepper

Instructions

- Start by preheating the oven until it reaches 400°F (200°C).
- Cut the chicken into small pieces. Chop or grate the peppers and onions.
- Mix all the ingredients, leaving a third of cheese in an already greased baking dish.
- Add the remaining cheese and bake for about 15 to 20 minutes or until golden brown.
- You can serve with greens dressed in olive oil.

Nutritional information:

Net carbs: 3% (10 g)

Fiber: 3 g

Fat: 77% (98 g)

Protein: 20% (57 g)

Kcal: 1148

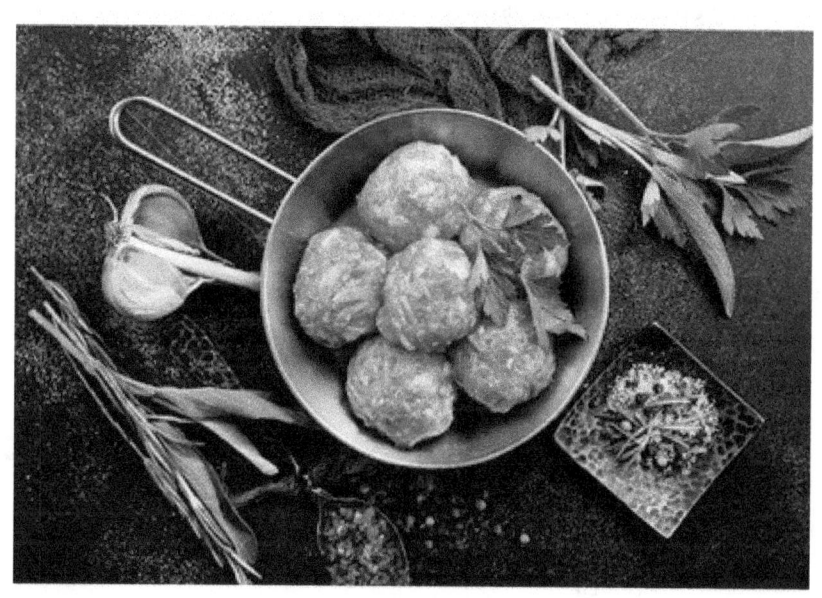

Chapter 10: Pork and Beef

Keto Pimiento Cheese Meatballs

They are simply delicious. They're good for both dinner and snacking.

Ingredients

Pimiento

Cheese

1/4 cup pimientos or pickled jalapeños

1/3 cup mayonnaise

1 pinch cayenne pepper

1 tablespoon Dijon mustard

1 egg

1 tablespoon chili powder or paprika powder

25 oz. ground beef

2 tablespoons butter, for frying

Salt and pepper

Instructions

- Mix all the ingredients in a large bowl and set aside for a few minutes.
- Add the egg and ground beef to the mixture. Mix properly using clean hands or a wooden spoon. Add salt and pepper to taste.
- Mold large meatballs and fry in a skillet with margarine or oil at medium-high heat until thoroughly cooked.
- You can serve with whatever side dish you desire, homemade

mayonnaise, and maybe a green salad.

Nutritional information:

Net carbs: 1% (1 g)

Fiber: 1 g

Fat: 73% (53 g)

Protein: 26% (42 g)

Kcal: 660

Classic Keto Hamburger

This is delicious and can be eaten with keto buns.

Ingredients

5 oz. cooked bacon

1 3/4 lbs. ground beef

2 oz. shredded lettuce

8 tablespoons mayonnaise

1 red onion

1 oz. olive oil or margarine, for frying

1 tomato

Salt and pepper

Ingredients for the keto hamburger buns

5 tablespoons ground psyllium husk powder

1 1/4 cups almond flour

3 eggs

1 1/4 cups boiling water

3 tablespoons baking powder

1 tablespoon sesame seeds

3 egg whites

2 tablespoons cold vinegar or white wine

Instructions

- Heat the oven to 350°F (175°C)
- Begin the cooking by preparing the hamburger buns. Mix the dry ingredients in a dry bowl.
- Boil the water and add it, the egg whites, and the vinegar to the bowl while mixing with a hand mixer for up to 30 seconds. Don't overmix the dough; make it as smooth as Play-Doh.
- Use moist hands to mold the dough into pieces of bread, one per serving. Sprinkle some sesame seeds over it. Ensure you create some space on the baking sheet to accommodate the buns when they double in size.
- Put on the lower rack in the oven and bake for about 50 to 60 minutes. Once you hear a slight sound when you tap the bottom of the buns, that's a sign that they are ready.

Preparing the hamburgers

While the bread is baking, you can prepare the condiments. Slice the onion and tomato thinly, shred the lettuce, and fry the bacon.

Mold the ground beef into single pieces of hamburger and grill or fry. Add some salt and pepper to taste when the hamburger is almost ready.

Cut the bread into halves and lavishly spread a good quantity of mayonnaise on both halves.

Make your hamburger the way you want it to taste.

Eat with coleslaw as a side for extra crunch.

Nutritional information:

Net carbs: 3% (6 g)

Fiber: 10 g

Fat: 76% (87 g)

Protein: 21% (54 g)

Kcal: 1067

Keto Ground Beans And Green Beans

This meal is a real wonder; it's affordable and simple to prepare. Perfect for dinner and yet fast food.

Ingredients

9 oz. fresh green beans

10 oz. ground beef

1/3 cup crème fraiche or mayonnaise (optional)

Salt and pepper

3 1/2 oz. margarine

Instructions

- Wash and trim the green beans.

- Heat a good amount of margarine with a frying pan that can hold both the green beans and the ground beef.
- Use high heat to brown the ground beef until it's almost ready and then add salt and pepper.
- Reduce the heat, add extra margarine, and fry the beans for about 5 minutes, using the same pan. You should stir the ground beef very often.
- Add salt and pepper to the beans. You can then serve the remaining margarine and add some crème fraiche or mayonnaise if you need more fat for satisfaction.
- You can make this meal using other low-carb veggies like asparagus, spinach, zucchini, or broccoli. Use your choice of spices to add more flavor to the vegetables, meat, and dip.

Nutritional information:

Net carbs: 3% (5 g)

Fiber: 3 g

Fat: 78% (60 g)

Protein: 19% (32 g)

Kcal: 694

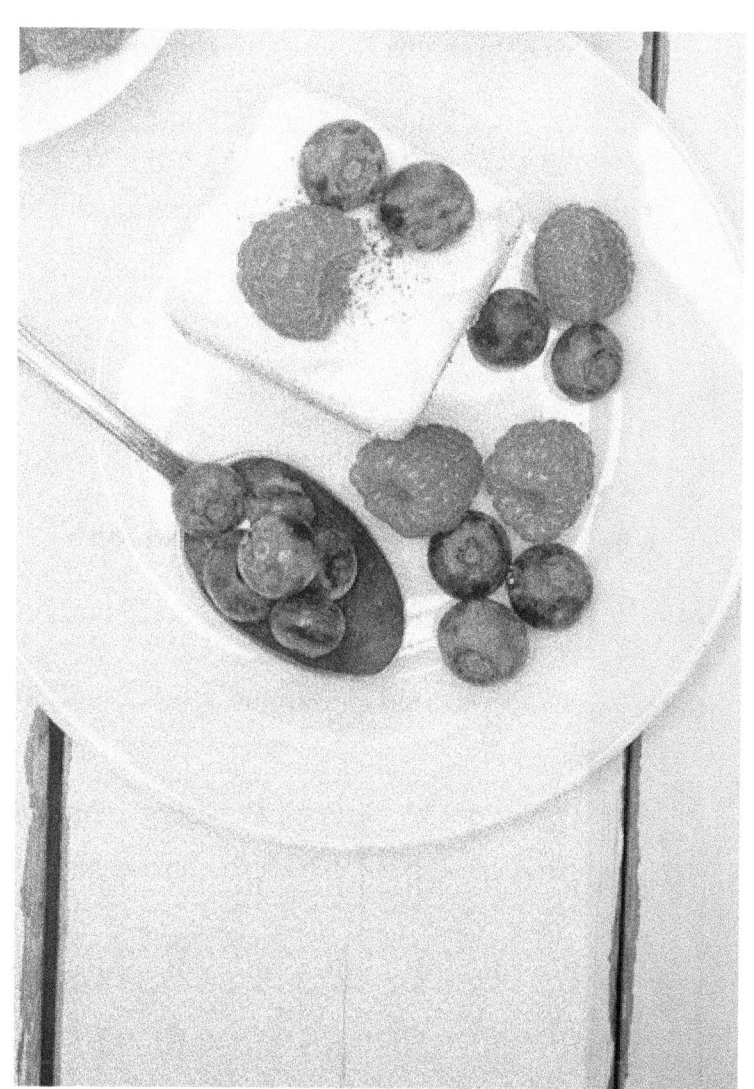

Chapter 11: Desserts and Treats

Pumpkin Spice Fat Bombs

Pumpkin is a natural choice for desserts, especially those that also include warm spices reminiscent of holiday pumpkin pie. Like its vegetable counterpart, carrots, the bright orange flesh of pumpkin indicates it is a stellar source of beta-carotene.

Pumpkin is also very high in vitamins A and C as well as potassium, making this pretty ingredient perfect for flushing toxins from your body and fighting cancer.

Ingredients

3 tablespoons chopped almonds

1/2 cup butter, at room temperature

1/3 cup pure pumpkin purée

1/2 cup cream cheese, at room temperature

4 drops liquid stevia

1/4 teaspoon ground nutmeg

1/2 teaspoon ground cinnamon

Instructions

- Line an 8-by-8-inch pan with parchment paper and set aside.
- In a small bowl, whisk the butter and cream cheese together until very smooth.
- Add the pumpkin purée and whisk until blended.
- Stir in the almonds, cinnamon, stevia, and nutmeg.
- Spoon the pumpkin mixture into the pan. Use a spatula or the back of a spoon to spread it evenly in the pan, then place in the freezer for about 1 hour.
- Cut into 16 pieces and store the fat bombs in a tightly sealed container in the freezer until ready to serve.

Nutritional information:

Net carbs: 5% (1 g)

Fiber: 0 g

Fat: 90% (9 g)

Protein: 5% (1 g)

Kcal: 87

Chocolate-Coconut Treats

Chocolate and coconut are a flawless combination often found in candy bars and many desserts. If you want a more elegant presentation, omit the coconut in step 3 and roll the semi-hardened chocolate mixture into balls instead of spreading in a pan. Then roll the balls in the shredded coconut and place the treats in the freezer to firm up completely.

Ingredients

¼ cup unsweetened cocoa powder

1/3 Cup coconut oil

Pinch sea salt

1/4 cup shredded unsweetened coconut

4 drops liquid stevia coconut

Instructions

- Line a 6-by-6-inch baking dish with parchment paper and set aside.
- In a small saucepan over low heat, stir together the coconut oil, cocoa, stevia, and salt for about 3 minutes.
- Stir in the coconut and press the mixture into the baking dish.
- Place the baking dish in the refrigerator until the mixture is hard, about 30 minutes.
- Cut into 16 pieces and store the treats in an airtight container in a cool place.

    For a more finished look, you can spoon the hot mixture into candy molds instead of a baking dish. Pop the molds in the refrigerator for 30 minutes or until firm and pop the treats out into a container.

Nutritional information:

Net carbs: 6% (1 g)

Fiber: 0 g

Fat: 88% (5 g)

Protein: 6% (1 g)

Kcal: 43

Almond Butter Fudge

Fudge should be smooth and dense with no grittiness or graininess. Since you won't be using granulated sugar for this treat, the chances of getting the wrong texture are greatly reduced. Almond butter is a stellar source of protein, vitamin E, iron, manganese, and fiber. If you are not a fan of this nut butter, peanut butter or cashew butter would also be delicious and creates the same tempting results.

Ingredients

1 cup coconut oil, at room temperature

1/4 cup heavy (whipping) cream

1 cup almond butter

10 drops liquid stevia

Pinch sea salt

Instructions

- Line a 6-by-6-inch baking dish with parchment paper and set aside.
- In a medium bowl, whisk together the heavy cream, almond butter, coconut oil, stevia, and salt until very smooth.
- Spoon the mixture into the baking dish and smooth the top with a spatula.
- Place the dish in the refrigerator until the fudge is firm, about 2

- hours.
- Cut into 36 pieces and store the fudge in an airtight container in the freezer for up to 2 weeks.

Nutritional information:

Net carbs: 5% (3 g)

Fiber: 1 g

Fat: 90% (22 g)

Protein: 5% (3 g)

Kcal: 204

Nutty Shortbread Cookies

Traditional shortbread has very few ingredients and is intensely buttery, slightly crumbly, and not too sweet. The nuts used here in place of flour create the desired texture and add a complex, pleasing flavor. These cookies will continue to cook on the baking sheets after you eat them out of the oven, so don't forget to transfer them to wire racks quickly to avoid over-browning.

Ingredients

1/2 cup butter, at room temperature, plus additional for greasing baking sheet

1 1/2 cups almond flour

1/2 cup granulated sweetener

1/2 cup ground hazelnuts

1 teaspoon alcohol-free pure vanilla extract

Pinch sea salt

Instructions

- In a medium bowl, cream together the sweetener, butter, and vanilla until well blended.

- Stir in the almond flour, ground hazelnuts, and salt until a firm dough is formed.
- Roll the dough into a 2-inch cylinder and wrap it in plastic wrap. Place the dough in the refrigerator for at least 30 minutes until firm.
- Preheat the oven to 350°F (175°C). Line a baking sheet with parchment paper and lightly grease the paper with butter; set aside.
- Unwrap the chilled cylinder, slice the dough into 18 cookies, and place the cookies on the baking sheet.
- Bake the cookies until firm and lightly browned, about 10 minutes.
- Allow the cookies to cool on the baking sheet for 5 minutes and then transfer them to a wire rack to cool completely.
- Process less expensive whole nuts in a food processor or blender rather than paying for a pre-ground product. Make sure you don't process the nuts in the appliance too long or you'll end up with nut butter.

Nutritional information:

Net carbs: 6% (2 g)

Fiber: 1 g

Fat: 85% (10 g)

Protein: 9% (3 g)

Kcal: 105

Vanilla-Almond Ice Pops

In childhood, nothing was better than a sweet treat on a hot summer day. This is a more elegant ice pop that can be enjoyed after a leisurely barbecue with friends. It features simple vanilla and coconut flavoring, which can be enhanced with cut fruit if you want a little more texture to the pop. Use inexpensive ice pop molds; they are easily found for a few dollars in most stores.

Ingredients

1 cup heavy (whipping) cream

2 cups almond milk

1 vanilla bean, halved lengthwise

1 cup shredded unsweetened coconut

Instructions

- Place a medium saucepan over medium heat and add the almond milk, heavy cream, and vanilla bean.
- Bring the liquid to a simmer and reduce the heat to low. Continue to simmer for 5 minutes.
- Remove the saucepan from the heat and let the liquid cool.
- Take the vanilla bean out of the liquid and use a knife to scrape the seeds out of the bean into the liquid.
- Stir in the coconut and divide the liquid between the ice pop molds.
- Freeze until solid, about 4 hours, and enjoy.

Nutritional information:

Net carbs: 10% (4 g)

Fiber: 2 g

Fat: 81% (15 g)

Protein: 9% (3 g)

Kcal: 166

Raspberry Cheesecake

Cheesecake is a sublime dessert experience: tart, sweet, and infinitely velvety on the tongue. This is a crust-free cheesecake featuring plump, ripe raspberries and a distinct vanilla undertone. You can use any type of berry, sliced peaches or plums, or even a tablespoon of cocoa powder to create gorgeous variations. Your imagination is the limit when you have a perfect cheesecake base to use in your experiments.

Ingredients

1/2 cup cream cheese, at room temperature

2/3 cup coconut oil, melted

6 eggs

3 tablespoons granulated sweetener

3/4 cup raspberries

1 teaspoon alcohol-free pure vanilla extract

1/2 teaspoon baking powder

Instructions

- Preheat the oven to 350°F (175°C). Line an 8-by-8-inch baking dish with parchment paper and set aside.
- In a large bowl, beat together the coconut oil and cream cheese until smooth.
- Beat in the eggs, scraping down the sides of the bowl at least once.
- Beat in the sweetener, vanilla, and baking powder until smooth.
- Spoon the batter into the baking dish and use a spatula to smooth out the top. Scatter the raspberries on top.
- Bake until the center is firm, about 25 to 30 minutes.
- Allow the cheesecake to cool completely before cutting into 12 squares.

  Any type of berry is delicious in this luscious treat, such as blueberries, strawberries, or blackberries. Whenever possible for your recipes, use seasonal local fruit for the best flavor and color.

Nutritional information:

Net carbs: 4% (3 g)

Fiber: 1 g

Fat: 85% (18 g)

Protein: 11% (6 g)

Kcal: 176

Calendar

Sunday	Monday	Tuesday	Wednesday	Thursday	Friday	Saturday
				1	2	3
4	5	6	7	8	9	10
11	12	13	14	15	16	17
18	19	20	21	22	23	24
25	26	27	28	29	30	31

Chapter 12: The 30-Day Meal Plan

12.1

The meal plan is meant to serve as a guide, so it's not compulsory you follow this, you can adjust it to fit your taste and schedule using the recipes earlier that were discussed in the previous chapters.

Some of the recipes are easy and straightforward to prepare while some others require early and proper planning, so put that into consideration as you start the diet.

12.2

Having a meal plan at the start of your diet gives you higher chances of success. A meal plan gives you a sense of direction. Many times, people give up because they don't have a good plan in place.

A meal plan in place means you have an idea of what you're eating as your next meal. This is key to achieving success as many people give up because they usually don't have a good meal plan in place.

The meal plan is what sustains you on the keto diet. Many out there are complaining about how they tried the diet for some time and because they weren't seeing any changes

DAY 1
Breakfast: Avocado and Eggs
Snack: Spinach-Blueberry Smoothie
Lunch: Cauliflower Cheddar Soup (leftovers)
Snack: Nutty Shortbread Cookies
Dinner: Baked Coconut Haddock and Brussels Sprouts Casserole

DAY 2
Breakfast: Lemon-Cashew Smoothie

Snack: Almond Butter Fudge

Lunch: BLT Salad

Snack: Bacon-Pepper Fat Bombs

Dinner: Roasted Pork Loin with Grainy Mustard Sauce and Golden Rosti

DAY 3

Breakfast: Peanut Butter Cup Smoothie

Snack: Walnut Herb-Crusted Goat Cheese

Lunch: Cauliflower-Cheddar Soup

Snack: Bacon-Cheese Deviled Eggs

Dinner: Lamb Leg with Sun-Dried Tomato Pesto (leftovers) and Sautéed Crispy Zucchini

DAY 4

Breakfast: Nut Medley Granola

Snack: Bacon-Cheese Deviled Eggs

Lunch: Chicken-Avocado Lettuce Wraps

Snack: Creamy Cinnamon Smoothie

Dinner: Lamb Leg with Sun-Dried Tomato Pesto and Cheesy Mashed Cauliflower

DAY 5

Breakfast: Nut Medley Granola

Snack: Smoked Salmon Fat Bombs

Lunch: Breakfast Bake

Snack: Almond Butter Fudge

Dinner: Chicken Bacon Burger and Portobello Mushroom Pizza

DAY 6

Breakfast: Berry Green Smoothie

Snack: Bacon-Pepper Fat Bombs

Lunch: Roasted Pork Loin with Grainy Mustard Sauce (leftovers)

Snack: Vanilla-Almond Ice Pops

Dinner: Turkey Meatloaf and Golden Rosti

DAY 7

Breakfast: Breakfast Bake

Snack: Creamy Cinnamon Smoothie

Lunch: Turkey Meatloaf (leftovers)

Snack: Nutty Shortbread Cookies

Dinner: Cheesy Garlic Salmon and Garlicky Green Beans

DAY 8

Breakfast: Peanut Butter Cup Smoothie

Snack: Crispy Parmesan Crackers

Lunch: BLT Salad

Snack: Smoked Salmon Fat Bombs

Dinner: Lamb Leg with Sun-Dried Tomato Pesto (leftovers) and Cheesy Mashed Cauliflower

DAY 9

Breakfast: Avocado and Eggs

Snack: Almond Butter Fudge

Lunch: Cauliflower-Cheddar Soup

Snack: Berry Green Smoothie

Dinner: Herb Butter Scallops and Pesto Zucchini Noodles

DAY 10

Breakfast: Nut Medley Granola

Snack: Vanilla-Almond Ice Pops

Lunch: Crab Salad-Stuffed Avocado

Snack: Chocolate-Coconut Treats

Dinner: Lamb Leg with Sun-Dried Tomato Pesto and Brussels Sprouts Casserole

DAY 11

Breakfast: Berry Green Smoothie

Snack: Nutty Shortbread Cookies

Lunch: Chicken-Avocado Lettuce Wraps

Snack: Crispy Parmesan Crackers

Dinner: Baked Coconut Haddock and Brussels Sprouts Casserole

DAY 12

Breakfast: Breakfast Bake

Snack: Queso Dip

Lunch: Roasted Pork Loin with Grainy Mustard Sauce (leftovers)

Snack: Almond Butter Fudge

Dinner: Lemon Butter Chicken and Sautéed Asparagus with Walnuts

DAY 13

Breakfast: Nut Medley Granola

Snack: Chicken-Avocado Lettuce Wraps

Lunch: Breakfast Bake

Snack: Raspberry Cheesecake with 1/4 cup whipped cream

Dinner: Turkey Meatloaf and Creamed Spinach

DAY 14

Breakfast: Lemon-Cashew Smoothie

Snack: Peanut Butter Mousse

Lunch: Cauliflower-Cheddar Soup (leftovers)

Snack: Chocolate-Coconut Treats

Dinner: Roasted Pork Loin with Grainy Mustard Sauce and Mushrooms with Camembert

DAY 15

Breakfast: Breakfast Bake

Snack: Almond Butter Fudge

Lunch: Chicken-Avocado Lettuce Wraps

Snack: Nutty Shortbread Cookies

Dinner: Lemon Butter Chicken and Sautéed Asparagus with Walnuts

DAY 16

Breakfast: Avocado and Eggs

Snack: Bacon-Pepper Fat Bombs

Lunch: Lemon-Cashew Smoothie

Snack: Almond Butter Fudge

Dinner: Baked Coconut Haddock and Brussels Sprouts Casserole

DAY 17

Breakfast: Avocado and Eggs

Snack: Crispy Parmesan Crackers

Lunch: Chicken-Avocado Lettuce Wraps

Snack: Queso Dip

Dinner: Turkey Meatloaf and Creamed Spinach

DAY 18

Breakfast: Berry Green Smoothie

Snack: Raspberry Cheesecake with 1/4 cup whipped cream

Lunch: BLT Salad

Snack: Crispy Parmesan Crackers

Dinner: Roasted Pork Loin with Grainy Mustard Sauce and Mushrooms with Camembert

DAY 19

Breakfast: Creamy Cinnamon Smoothie

Snack: Chocolate-Coconut Treats

Lunch: Cauliflower-Cheddar Soup

Snack: Vanilla-Almond Ice Pops

Dinner: Herb Butter Scallops and Pesto Zucchini Noodles

DAY 20

Breakfast: Peanut Butter Cup Smoothie

Snack: Almond Butter Fudge

Lunch: Crab Salad-Stuffed Avocado

Snack: Nutty Shortbread Cookies

Dinner: Baked Coconut Haddock and Brussels Sprouts Casserole

DAY 21

Breakfast: Lemon-Cashew Smoothie

Snack: Berry Green Smoothie

Lunch: Roasted Pork Loin with Grainy Mustard Sauce (leftovers)

Snack: BLT Salad

Dinner: Turkey Meatloaf and Creamed Spinach

DAY 22

Breakfast: Avocado and Eggs

Snack: Bacon-Pepper Fat Bombs

Lunch: Turkey Meatloaf (leftovers)

Snack: Walnut Herb-Crusted Goat Cheese

Dinner: Roasted Pork Loin with Grainy Mustard Sauce and Golden Rosti

DAY 23

Breakfast: Creamy Cinnamon Smoothie

Snack: Nutty Shortbread Cookies

Lunch: Crab Salad-Stuffed Avocado

Snack: Berry Green Smoothie

Dinner: Roasted Pork Loin with Grainy Mustard Sauce and Mushrooms with Camembert

DAY 24

Breakfast: Breakfast Bake

Snack: Berry Green Smoothie

Lunch: Chocolate-Coconut Treats

Snack: BLT Salad

Dinner: Herb Butter Scallops and Pesto Zucchini Noodles

DAY 25

Breakfast: Peanut Butter Cup Smoothie

Snack: Nutty Shortbread Cookies

Lunch: Creamy Cinnamon Smoothie

Snack: Vanilla-Almond Ice Pops

Dinner: Turkey Meatloaf and Creamed Spinach

DAY 26

Breakfast: Berry Green Smoothie

Snack: BLT Salad

Lunch: Cauliflower-Cheddar Soup

Snack: Raspberry Cheesecake with 1/4 cup whipped cream

Dinner: Lamb Leg with Sun-Dried Tomato Pesto (leftovers) and Cheesy Mashed Cauliflower

DAY 27

Breakfast: Creamy Cinnamon Smoothie

Snack: Crispy Parmesan Crackers

Lunch: Crab Salad-Stuffed Avocado

Snack: Queso Dip

Dinner: Lemon Butter Chicken and Sautéed Asparagus with Walnuts

DAY 28

Breakfast: Crispy Parmesan Crackers

Snack: Nutty Shortbread Cookies

Lunch: Chicken-Avocado Lettuce Wraps

Snack: Almond Butter Fudge

Dinner: Lemon Butter Chicken and Sautéed Asparagus with Walnuts

DAY 29

Breakfast: Creamy Cinnamon Smoothie

Snack: Chocolate-Coconut Treats

Lunch: Cauliflower-Cheddar Soup

Snack: Vanilla-Almond Ice Pops

Dinner: Herb Butter Scallops and Pesto Zucchini Noodles

DAY 30

Breakfast: Lemon-Cashew Smoothie

Snack: Peanut Butter Mousse

Lunch: Cauliflower-Cheddar Soup (leftovers)

Snack: Chocolate-Coconut Treats

Dinner: Roasted Pork Loin with Grainy Mustard Sauce and Mushrooms with Camembert

12.3

How to use the meal plan:

- You should start thinking and planning for your meals at least 3 days before. Don't just choose recipes in an undeliberate manner, it is smart to actually choose recipes you're a bit familiar alongside the new ones. This way you won't feel overwhelmed.
- Using the guideline, you should have a daily consumption of about

1500 to 1900 calories. If you don't have an idea how many calories you are meant to eat, check using an online macro calculator. In a case where you need more calories than what is available in the meal plan, you can switch any of the meals for one with higher calories or you can also add more oil or an ingredient while cooking.

- This meal plan is designed for one person. This means that if you want to use them for more people, all you need to do is multiply the quantity of ingredients by the number of people.
- Since some of the recipes in the meal plan might not be meals you used to cook prior to this time, you should shop for your ingredients earlier than when you need them. You could start shopping over the weekend. You don't have to take a very big list to the store for shopping, simply start by planning for the first week.
- Prepare the ingredients that need to prepped beforehand.
- If you're on a very strict keto diet, ensure you tweak this meal plan to make it work for you.
- If you are allergic to any ingredient, ensure you replace them with other low-carb substitutes.

Your Quick-Start Action Step:

Draft your meal plan and find out how much it will cost you to prepare the recipes in your meal plan. This is an important part of becoming successful with the diet.

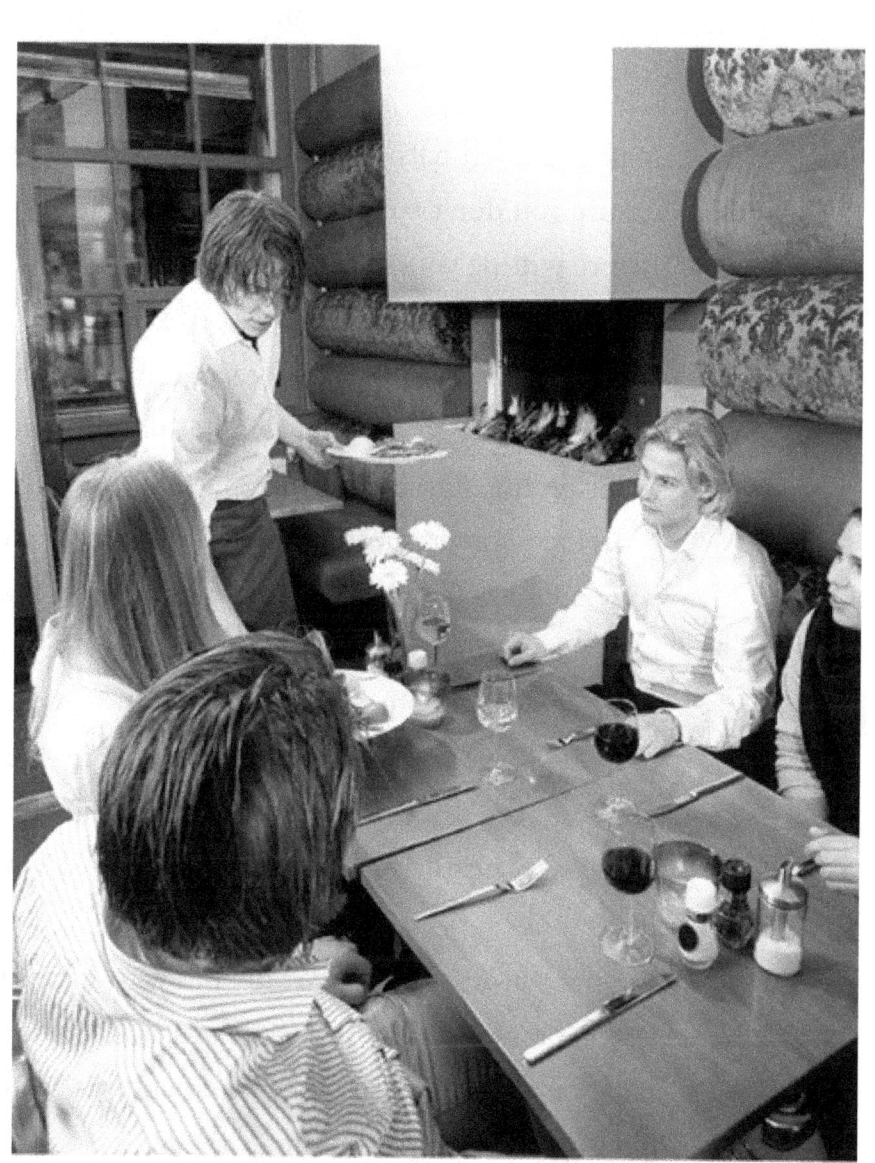

Chapter 13: How to Dine Out with the Keto Diet

This is a guide to ensure that even though you are having dinner anywhere, you still maintain your keto diet. It is very possible to obtain low-carb food anywhere. Below are some tips to help with enjoying a delicious meal anywhere and yet not compromising your diet lifestyle:

- Make a sacred oath – this is arguably the most important tip to ensure you don't compromise your diet lifestyle while dining out. Before putting yourself in such a situation, make a commitment to strictly avoid the big offenders (carbs).
- Ditch the starch – avoid the bread, the pasta, the potatoes, and the rice. It's better to keep all temptation off your plate by not even ordering the starchy food in the first place. If after such careful ordering your order still arrives with a starchy side, then weigh your options. If you are confident and sure that you will leave it untouched, then you can go on with feasting, but if you feel the craving to "just taste some," then you should request for your meal to be replaced with something that contains no starch, and if you don't want to draw unnecessary attention to yourself then you can find a way to discard the unwanted pieces of your food in the nearest bin.
- Embrace healthy fat –take fate into your hands whenever you visit a restaurant; you can request extra butter and let it melt on your meat or veggie. When your meal contains salad, you can request olive oil and vinegar dressing.
- Pay more attention to protein, vegetables and fats; it is important to focus on the healthy food, as long as your mind is fixated on them, your cravings for the other unsafe foods will be reduced. It is relatively easy to obtain healthy fats to add to your plates. Example

of these include butter, olive oil, and sour cream. You can request them if you don't see them.

- Be very careful when choosing your drink; some drinks are perfectly fine and completely safe, for example; tea, coffee, or water. Some alcoholic beverages are also fine, like dry wine, light beer, or champagne.

- Watch out for condiments and sauces; some sauces have a very high fat content, for example, like Béarnaise sauce, while others consist mostly of carbs, like ketchup. If you are not certain of the content of the sauce you're given, then ask, and avoid it if it consists mostly of sugar or flour.

- Is dessert really necessary – you don't need to order dessert unless it's really required; you can just stick with a cup of coffee while others can finish their sweets. If you feel your coffee is hardly satisfying then adding butter or cream to it is enough to satiate your need.

- Be patient – get into the dinner conversation, remember to stay hydrated, and enjoy your tea or coffee. Usually, being on a keto diet means that it may eat a bit of a while before you are satisfied; however, don't give in to the need to eat in overdrive—this won't help if you're trying to lose weight. Give it some time; you might eventually feel satisfied.

- Ensure you ease the edge your hunger before leaving home; it is only safe to eat a fatty snack before leaving for the party. You can pick olives, nuts or cheese, any of these are good choices. This makes it much easier to say no to the big offenders (starchy foods).

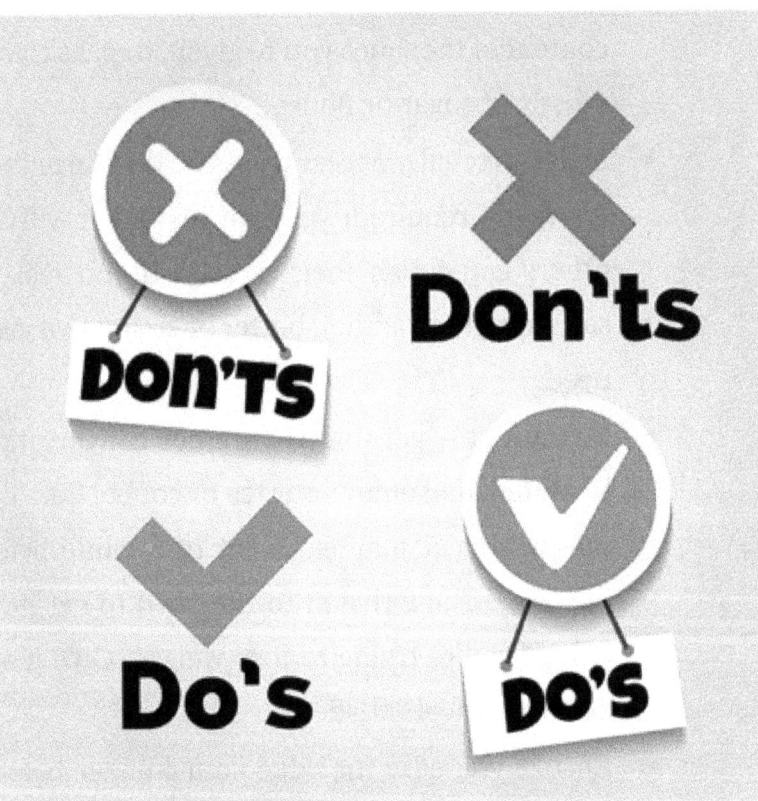

Chapter 14: Mistakes To Avoid When On A Keto Diet

Being on a ketogenic diet is not so easy. It requires a whole lot of commitment and focus since it entails you changing your normal routine. Your body is going to undergo an internal change, and your normal daily activities will have to change too. Many people, upon being on a keto diet, do not see results as fast as they hope, while others really love it. What makes the difference is certain common mistakes that people make when beginning a ketogenic diet. This is fine, as no one is really perfect and mistakes do happen. We must all learn that mistakes are to be learned from in other to avoid making them again.

Below are some of the common mistakes that people make when staying on a keto diet. This will help you avoid these mistakes as you continue on your keto diet journey.

- Doing keto as a quick fix – the keto diet is not a quick fix to solve your body issues. It is a new way of life that you have to stick to and be consistent with in order to see results. You may notice some fast changes as soon as you start a keto diet but this doesn't mean you can go right back to your old eating habits and still expect these changes to remain. It's very likely you'll go back to how you were before, with all those changes completely lost. Do not expect that such changes are going to be permanent just by being loyal to keto for a couple of months.
- Worrying too much over the scale – it is true that one of the benefits of being on a keto diet is that it helps with weight loss, helping burn stored-up body fat. However, it is important to note that this is a process that takes time and being too fixated and obsessed over your weight is going to make it look longer and harder. Frequently checking your weight is not going to

help, whether multiple times a day or even daily. You just have to trust that since you are doing things the right way, then results are bound to come, and that staying off carbs and hitting your macros daily is going to make your weight come off. Constant checking of your weight only puts a heavy weight on your mind and leaves you discouraged. Significant changes occur over multiple weeks or months. It is advisable to only check your weight once a week.

- Fear of fats – it sounds like an oxymoron to say that you actually have to eat fat to lose fat, but this is true and actually works. When staying on a keto diet, it is quite important to eat a large amount of fat to ensure your body reaches the set goal. Fat is not bad for you when on a keto diet, and when you calculate your macros and discover the large amount of fat you have to consume, don't be afraid. Fat must contribute up to 75 percent of your diet when on a ketogenic diet; this is how you can be successful with it. So understanding that this amount of fat is going to help, will make you not afraid but rather help you in embracing high fat consumption.

- Consuming the wrong type of fat – eating fat when on a keto diet is very essential, but you must ensure that you're eating the right type of fat. There are good fats to embrace and bad fats to avoid when starting a keto diet; don't just assume that since you require a large fat content in your diet then all fats are good for you. The bad fats are the processed fats—they are present in processed vegetable oils. Therefore, cooking with these oils is a big fat no. The good fats that you need are the monounsaturated fats, naturally occurring trans-fats, saturated fats, and the polyunsaturated fats. Getting these types of fats is easy. The good fats are present in foods like avocados, walnuts, eggs, butter, etc. When these are added to your diet, you'll realize than not only are you meeting the fat requirements of your body but you're also sticking with the good fats.

- Consuming excess protein in your diet – some do not see this as a problem when staying on a keto diet; they see this as a substitute for their low-carb diet. However, it is important to note that having too much protein in your diet will have certain undesirable effects on your body. When an excess amount of protein is consumed, the body only utilizes the amount it requires while the remaining is converted to fat, storing it up in the body; this is bad as reducing weight is what we want to achieve and not the exact opposite. It is very simple to avoid this: all you need do is simply to focus more on your macros so as not to have an excessive intake of anything.

- Not drinking enough water – when doing the keto diet, one of the internal changes that your body undergoes is loss of body fluids. To counter this, it is very important to stay hydrated by drinking a lot of water. When you're not staying hydrated, your body is going to respond by storing a lot of fat; again, this is bad as reducing weight is what we want to achieve and not the exact opposite. When you lose body fluids and electrolytes when on a keto diet, it can easily be replenished by consuming a large quantity of water. This will also help your body organs function properly and your body work effectively. Some individuals aren't comfortable with drinking a lot of water daily but this is something that has to be strictly followed if you want to see the changes that you desire. Usually, one gallon of water per day is recommended.

- Not having enough sleep – when your body begins to enter a state of ketosis and fat becomes your body's primary source of energy (as is usually the case when one is on a keto diet), it is normal that your body doesn't get as much sleep as before when you were still following your old eating habits. You therefore need to try, as much as possible, to get the right amount of sleep that you require. You need sleep, and getting the right amount is important, as not getting the right amount will affect the overall functioning of your body. When you get the right amount of sleep, it enables your body to cope with the numerous changes it undergoes as a result of being on a keto diet.

- Eating the same thing all the time – when on a keto diet, since you're restricted in the amounts of carb you can consume, it may give you the idea that you are also restricted in the number of recipes you can have as well. Because of this, some people seem to eat a monotonous meal, eating the same things all the time. When you mix things up properly, you will discover that your meal can actually be quite enjoyable. This will help in being consistent with staying on a ketogenic diet and not being discouraged; it allows you to want to go further with the diet as it keeps your morale high. It is okay to add in some low-carb vegetables to your diet every once in a while. You should ensure to keep your taste buds excited so even your favorite meal doesn't begin to taste bland due to eating it too often and you begin to get sick of it.

- Using others as a yardstick for yourself – this is a mental mistake but with a large effect on whether you are consistent with the keto diet or give up too quickly. It is a part of human nature to compare yourself with others; people love doing it and everyone does it. When on a ketogenic diet, you can't afford to compare yourself with others; your focus should be on your body and no one else as otherwise it will be like signing your own death warrant. The response of everyone's body to the diet differs with individuals; this means that people are going to experience changes in their body at different times and at different rates from yours. So simply focus more on your own body changes and trust that, since you're doing the right thing, your weight loss will come and you will reach your goal.

Most of these mistakes are easily avoided; some of them are physical while some are mostly mental. The mental ones are the hardest to avoid. Once you notice that you have made any of these mistakes just ensure that you take a step back, evaluate the situation, find out where the mistake came from, determine how it can be solved, and get right back to things.

Bonus Chapter: Other Types of the Keto Diet

15.1

The focus of this book is on the standard keto diet, however, there are other types of diets out there. Your goal and activity level will determine what type of ketogenic diet is best for you. You may have to try the different types out to find out which works well for you. There are other types namely; the Targeted, Cyclical and the High Protein ketogenic diet. The Targeted Ketogenic Diet is best for keeping up with exercise performance, energizing your muscles with a good amount of glucose during exercise. For someone who wants to try the targeted ketogenic diet, you should consume about 25 to 50 grams of net carbs up to 30 minutes or an hour before exercise, and then follow the standard ketogenic diet every other time. The targeted variant is best for two categories of people; people who require carbs for energy during exercise but cannot afford to have long loads of carb that the cyclical ketogenic diet offers, individuals who are just starting an exercise program and cannot afford to do the required amount of exercise to fully optimize a cyclical diet. However, people who have not tried the standard diet for at least one or two months are advised to not try this diet.

The Cyclical Ketogenic Diet combines the standard keto diet with carb loading days. It is usually used by people who have more intense exercise activities for example athletes and bodybuilders, this is because to optimize their performance during training, high volume and intensity is required. This diet makes it almost possible for them to be at their best while engaging in such voluminous and intense exercise. However, it is not recommended for people who are not well adapted to keto yet.

The High Protein Ketogenic Diet requires increasing the intake of protein. It's best for older people who stand high risks of muscle breakdown or people who need more protein to protect muscle mass like bodybuilders. It is equally a great choice for people who show signs of being deficient in protein. Such signs include thinning hair or loss or muscle. Individuals with kidney diseases and those who want to get on the keto diet for therapeutic reasons should not go on the high protein diet.

15.2 Each of the other types of the ketogenic diet comes with their benefits and are discussed shortly below.

Benefits of the Targeted Ketogenic Diet

While on the targeted keto diet, you can perform highly intense activities and yet not have to be out of ketosis for long periods of time. In other words, it increases energy levels for athletes and people who do strenuous exercises.

Going on the targeted keto diet can also be helpful to athletes in that it boosts the insulin level which prevents muscle break down and rather promotes muscle growth.

Benefits of the High Protein Ketogenic Diet

The high protein keto diet is helpful for achieving greater results with weight loss, this is also linked with the fact that it reduces hunger level. It has equally been proven to helpful in managing diabetes because it improves glycemic control in patients who have type-2 diabetes.

Benefits of the Cyclical Ketogenic Diet

The cyclical keto diet uses anabolic "growth" hormones like insulin to help athletes gain muscle as well as replenish the glycogen available in the body to enable them lift heavier weights.

The cyclical keto diet has also been proven to be helpful in restoring adrenals and revitalizing the thyroid.

15.3 Take some time and do a study on each of the types of the keto diet mentioned here. There's quite a volume of information available online about them, go online and read up.

Ketogenic Diet Conversion Tables

Liquid Volumes		
Ml	U.S.	Fl oz.
15	1 tbsp	½
30	1/8 c	1
60	1/4 c	2
118	1/2 c	4
177	3/4 c	6
237	1 c	8
355	1 1/2 c	12
474	2 c	16
710	3 c	24
746	4 c	32

Dry weights	
Grams	Oz – lb
28	1
57	2
85	3
113	4 oz – 1/4 lb

151	1/3 lb
227	8 oz – 1/2 lb
302	2/3 lb
340	12 oz – 3/4 lb
454	1 lb
907	2 lb

OVEN TEMPERATURES	
Celsius	Fahrenheit
140°	285°
150°	300°
160°	320°
170°	338°
180°	356°
200°	392°
220°	425°
225°	437°

Conclusion

Thank you again for owning this book!

I hope this book was able to help you to fully grasp what the ketogenic diet is all about. In order to be successful with the diet, the next step is to dutifully execute what you have learned in the book, especially the chapter about the guidelines for getting on the diet.

Thank you and good luck!

Keto Meal Prep for Beginners

Your Essential Ketogenic Diet Easy Meal Plan to Save Time & Money for Long-Term Weight Loss, Eating Better and Healthy Living (PLUS: Easy Meal Prep Ideas on a Budget)

Amy Maria Adams

Table of Contents

Introduction:

Chapter 1: Getting Started with Keto Meal Prep Plan

Chapter 2: How to Begin Meal Prepping

Chapter 3: Easy Steps to Meal Prepping

Chapter 4: Simple Go-To Recipes to Start

Chapter 5: The Main Recipes

Chapter 6: Keto Meal Prep on a Budget

Chapter 7: Keto Meal Prep for Weight Loss

Chapter 8: Keto Meal Prep—Mistakes to Avoid

Bonus Chapter: Money-Savings Tips When Shopping

Conclusion

Introduction:

It is unfortunate to say, but sometimes we are so busy to think of what we want or should eat, let alone what we should cook. It is not very easy to eat healthy foods if you lead a busy life unless you have everything planned. *Deciding what to eat every day can, sadly, be a source of stress.* What you will cook for dinner or what you will eat for breakfast or lunch can get tiring, especially if you are on a healthy lifestyle.

Now, imagine for someone who is on a diet such as the keto diet, which demands that you have to eat particular foods for the right nutrition to power your body with sufficient energy! While many of us aspire to live healthy lifestyles and set goals to eat healthy, it is never easy following through, and consistency is a big problem. In fact, it is something as simple as having the right meals to eat, which makes many of us fall off the wagon. This is why meal prepping is a great concept for those on the ketogenic diet.

When you're busy navigating through your daily life, the thought of cooking all of your own meals at home can sometimes feel impossible. Not to mention warding off temptations at restaurants. And let's face it—time is the number-one "make or break" factor when it comes to deciding on a meal.

Those who are on a ketogenic diet know all too well that *it can be a tricky affair getting the food you like at an affordable price and which will not take a long time to prepare after a long day or even on those days when you just feel off.* Keto meal prepping ensures that you have the food as per your diet all the time—the question of what you should eat will never arise.

For somebody who may be wondering what a ketogenic diet is or someone who is looking for a great dieting option, *the keto diet focuses on foods that will get your body into a metabolic state of called ketosis, where the body burns fat for energy instead of carbs. In other words, you will be on a high-fat, low-carb diet to achieve weight loss or other dieting goals.*

The idea is based on the fact that most weight gain and fat accumulation in the body is as a result of high carbs intake. Carbohydrates are converted into glycogen and fat by the body. The glycogen is stored in the muscles, and the leftover converted carbs are stored as fat.

When the body is starved of new carbs, it burns up the glycogen stored in the muscles. Once exhausted, the body resorts to the fat reservoir for energy. It is for this reason that the ketogenic diet is so popular and is the most recommended diet for weight loss. It is essentially weight loss without opting out of some foods. You can eat virtually anything you want as long as it fits into the diet.

Ketosis has proven to have a variety of health benefits, which include weight loss, blood sugar regulation, disease management (diabetes, high blood pressure, cholesterol issues, etc.), and enhanced mental performance. Ketosis starves your body of carbohydrates, which the liver converts to glucose—reduced glucose means the body burns fat for energy.

Back to the topic at hand. *Meal prepping simply means preparing whole meals ahead of schedule so that they are available for you to eat when the time comes.* This concept is ideal for the busy lifestyle and has gained popularity with people for the amazing time-saving benefits and other benefits, which we will discuss later in this book.

Apart from having ready meals, this concept ensures that you eat reduces portion to help you reach your dieting goals. No more fast food because prepping guarantees that you eat more nutritious meals and no more late-night meals because you always have a ready dish.

The good thing about meal prepping is that you customize it to fit your availability and needs. There is no standard method of doing it. Choose the day to prep your meals and switch it if you have to.

What about if you are reading this and you are not on a keto diet? Well, meal prepping is still something you should consider for the many benefits on offer. Everyone wants an easier life; therefore, meal planning can be adopted by all of us. Meal prep is not only for those on a keto diet; it can be adapted to fit any diet and lifestyle to guarantee that you will have a meal ready for you ahead of time.

By the end of this book, you will be well informed about meal prepping in general but, more specifically, keto meal prep. This book will cover the following:

- How to get started on keto prep meal plan
- Information on how to begin prepping
- Easy steps to meal prepping
- Simple breakfast, lunch, dinner, desserts, and snack keto recipes for beginners or anyone who wants a quick-fix meal
- Main keto recipes
- Keto meal prepping on a budget
- Meal prepping for weight loss
- Money-saving tips
- Measurement conversions

Meal prepping will simplify your life, save you a lot of time and money, and ensure that you live the healthy lifestyle you want by keeping you on track as far as eating healthy meals is concerned.

The answer to eating what you want affordably and without putting so much time and energy into cooking is meal prepping, and we shall give you great insights and share with you some great recipes to start you off. Enjoy this introduction to meal prepping, the great recipes, and many other tips.

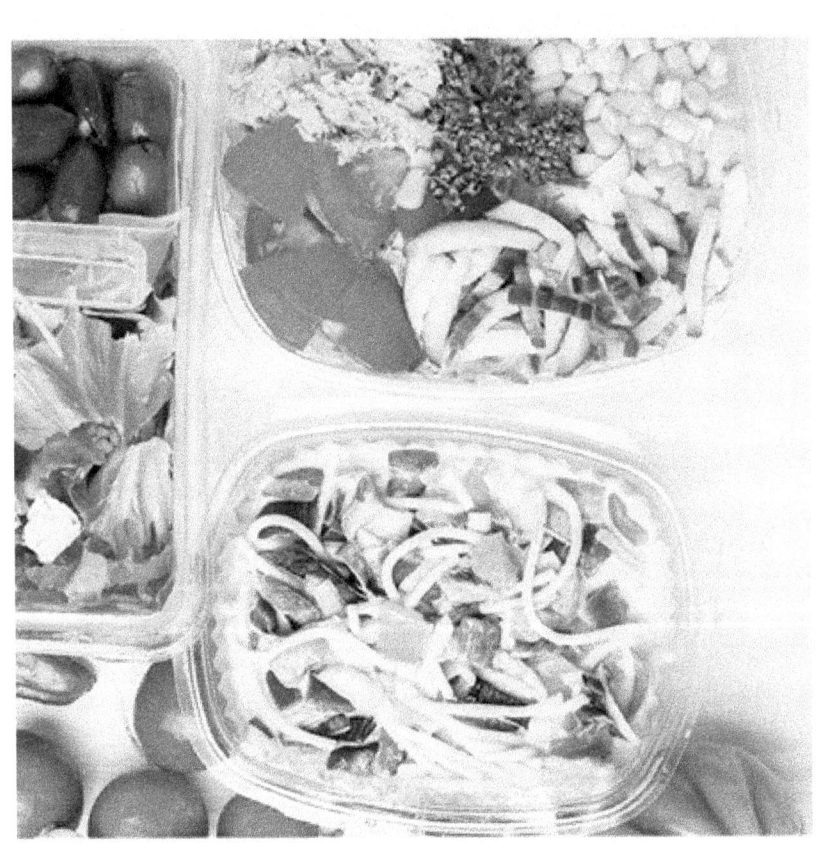

Chapter 1: Getting Started with Keto Meal Prep Plan

1.1 Definition of Keto Meal Prep Plan

We have touched on the meaning of a meal prep plan in the introduction and stated that it means to prepare meals in advance. *For the ketogenic diet, meal planning can be defined more specifically to mean preparing full meals in advance using keto approved ingredients, calories, and recipes so that you have meals ready to eat that meet the requirements of keto*, usually for a week.

The common and most convenient keto meal prep plan runs for a week. In other words, you will prepare meals for a whole week in advance on a designated day. Think about it, in one week, you will need twenty-one meals if you take three meals a day as you should. Thinking of the over-twenty meals daily or at mealtime is hard and is even more exhausting when you have to factor in the nutrition values of every meal because of the keto diet.

Keto meal planning is the way to solve the problem of cooking time, which can be hard to come by during the week, and will ensure that you eat the correct nutrients. More importantly, it is a flexible process that is owned by everyone in his or her own way so that one's needs, preferences, and schedule are conveniently accommodated.

Why You Need a Keto Meal Prep Plan

You well know that a keto diet requires certain amounts of nutrients, mainly carbohydrates, fat, and proteins per meal. Without proper planning, you can never eat right if you are on keto. Therefore, meal prepping ensures that you reach and maintain your dietary goals throughout the week by preventing you from making bad choices during the week.

Remember, for every meal you eat on a keto diet, you need a calorie breakdown as of 5% carbs, 75% fat, and 20% protein. How can you possibly achieve or ensure this every time without effective planning? Keto meal prep planning makes it possible to allocate one day to cook all the foods you will eat throughout the week and use the time you would otherwise spend cooking or thinking of what to cook on other things. A time-saver!

By doing all that planning for the whole week in one go, you reduce the stress of figuring out what to eat each day. You also save a lot of time, because you are not starting from scratch each day.

Meal prep will allow you to tailor-make meals to meet your keto needs. It is important to keep in mind that it is a process that will take time to learn but will simplify your routine if you stick to it.

Reasons for Keto Meal Prep Planning

Motivation alone is not enough for dieting or losing weight because you will never be motivated every time. There are times when your motivation will be shaken. However, researchers have found that planning is a better factor for dieting and weight-loss success.

Ninety-one percent of participants who planned and scheduled to work out did so at least once a week while only 35% of the study group who did not schedule a workout managed to exercise at least once a week, according to a study carried in the *British Journal of Health Psychology*. Planning ahead helps you to get things done.

Moreover, there are other benefits to meal planning, which include the following:

- Less stress and time deciding what to eat
- Saves time and money

- Helps you achieve dieting needs

1.2 How This Book Is Organized

Now that you have a better understanding of what keto meal prep planning is and why it is important, let us have an overview of what is in this book. This chapter will give you an idea of how long it takes to prep meals, the benefits of keto meal planning, and steps to get you ready for meal planning.

Further ahead in the book, there will be chapters on how to begin meal prepping, easy steps for meal prepping in detail, simple go-to recipes and main keto recipes, how to do keto meal prepping on a budget.

Additionally, the remainder of the book covers meal prepping for weight loss and mistakes to avoid when doing keto meal prepping. You will get a bonus chapter on money-saving tips to help you when shopping and a section on measurements conversions so that you get your nutrients and ingredients right.

Every chapter has a "Quick Start Action Step" section to guide you on the immediate actions to take for keto meal prep planning.

1.3 How Long Does It Take to Meal-Prep?

To be honest and objective, the duration you take for meal prepping will depend on you and for a variety of reasons, the main one being your preferences and speed. There are other things you need to do, like shopping for the ingredients you will need for your meals. However, *generally, it takes about an hour to cook meal preps for a week.*

The best time to plan and prep your keto meals would be a Saturday or Sunday, when most of us have a bit of a break from the rigors of work. Shopping in the afternoon is a good idea because you will not have to deal with the morning rush, keeping in mind that part of the reason why we are prepping is to reduce stress. You should be as relaxed and organized as possible with shopping.

Therefore, the best time to plan or decide the meals for the week would be Saturday morning before you go shopping. That means that you will have a designated time on Sunday to prep your dishes. The key to getting meal planning and prepping right is to pick a time that will be devoid of distraction or interruptions so that you can use the hour you have for cooking efficiently and optimally.

A distraction-free meal planning session is especially important for those who are starting out on keto meal prep planning. Once you are accustomed to the process, planning and prepping times will be reduced considerably. Find the best times that work for you.

A ketogenic diet requires prepping and planning because if you do not get the meals right, you will destabilize the body chemistry. To ease the process of keto meal prep, start with a week's meal plan, pick out the dishes you want for every one of the three meals per day. From the meals you have chosen, you will draw a detailed shopping list ahead of the shopping time so that you will spend as little time as possible buying them and have enough time for preparation.

The ketogenic diet meal prep plan is ideal for the busy person on the ketogenic diet who hardly ever has enough time to prepare his or her meals. If you leave for work early and are back home to sleep most of the week and you are on the keto diet, there is no better option to ensure that you keep on track despite your hectic schedule.

1.4 The Benefits of a Keto Diet Meal Prep Plan

- *It eliminates the temptation to eat off-diet.*

    Remember that you are on a diet. The keto diet is calories- and nutrients-specific, such that if you falter, you are likely to destabilize your body chemistry and reverse the gains you have made.

Keto meal prepping eliminates the temptation to eat fast food or any other meals that are not healthy since you have your meals prepared beforehand. With meal planning and prepping, the foods you eat will meet your dietary needs because they are well thought out, planned, and prepped in advance. All you will need to do is warm the food and eat it.

- *Keto meal planning and prepping saves time.*

Meal planning and prepping will save you time all round. You save time with shopping since you have a list of everything you want early enough. You save time with cooking since the ingredients are prepared early, and you save time on deciding what to eat. Consequently, you have more time to assign to other things, like spending time with family and friends, pursuing a hobby, or beating a deadline at work. You save a lot of time you would have spent cooking, shopping, and deciding meals.

- *Grocery shopping is made easy.*

Meal planning ensures that you know beforehand what you will require for your meals so that you do not leave out anything from your grocery shopping list or struggle to list items down at the last minute. The best way of detailing your shopping list is by sectionalizing the items into the various food categories, such as dairy, grains, fats, fruits, frozen foods, proteins, and veggies.

Always try to get a new food item each week for each category. If you bought tilapia last week for protein, get salmon this week. If you bought broccoli, get cauliflower this week. The list of items you buy must take into account the ketogenic diet nutritional requirement.

- *It makes meal decision-making easier and reduces stress.*

As many of you may know, settling on what to eat every day three times a week can be difficult and stressful. With keto meal prepping and planning, this problem will be completely eliminated because you do not have to make the decision every day—the decision about what to eat is made once for the whole week. The time you spend preparing your meals is significantly reduced because everything is planned ahead.

The stress that comes with deciding meals and keeping up with the requirements of your keto diet regime will also fizzle away with meal prepping. You will have a calmer and healthier mental predisposition and keep stress-related health problems at bay.

- *Keto meal prep planning saves money.*

Buying food items for your cooking in bulk saves you a lot of money. No impulse buying, no cases of buying the wrong ingredients because you will know exactly what to buy in advance. Pricing food items ahead brings in the effective element of cost control through portion control. You save money because you will not be eating out every time and will be buying items at a bargain.

Additionally, you will know the right quantities to buy, which will save you from the financial losses incurred through wastes, especially when you buy more than you need and have to throw away what is left or watch it go bad. You also save money by making fewer trips to the shop.

- *It gives you total control of what you eat and the calorie intake.*

Advance food planning and preparation gives you total control of your keto diet, enabling the consumption of the right calories and keto macros balance. The chances of you eating foods that are not recommended or going above the recommended calories are closely managed or eliminated.

You know too well that controlling what you eat, the portion, and your calorie intake is important for dieting and weight loss. Keto meal prepping will keep you within the right measures and will help you to attain ketosis for a healthy, efficient body.

- *It helps with hunger management.*

Hunger pangs are mainly triggered by predetermined mealtimes by habit. When the time comes when you normally eat dinner, you are likely to feel hungry. Keto meal prepping and planning will help you manage hunger by ensuring that you have the dish ready for the respective meal. Eating at the right time is also important to maintain the right ketosis metabolic balance.

- *You get time to do other things.*

Whether you want to call it multitasking or getting time for other things, keto meal prepping will get that for you. The many hours you have from not cooking and preparing meals can be used for other activities, which will improve your performance and productivity in other areas of your life.

This is the ideal option for those with a busy life and an in tray that is always full. You want a meal plan in the first place because of the time factor. You are busy and would prefer getting more done within the often short time that is available to you.

Even with the meal prepping process, you will be able to have multiple meals cooking because as something is baking in the oven, you could have another dish simmering on one burner, another stew on a different burner, and another burner frying another keto recipe, all within the prep time!

- *It will bring variety to your meals.*

Keto meal prepping ensures that you have a variety of healthy foods every weekly cycle. By alternating products within every food category, you cannot get bored with what you eat because of the variety at your disposal. As we said under the point of grocery shopping, you can eat different vegetables every day of the week or for every meal.

- *It will help you to lose weight.*

    Planning ketogenic meals in advance is key to weight loss. You will have the portions right, and the calorie intake will be as recommended. Consistency with the meals will help you to lose weight quickly.

Accordingly, this book is a great resource for those who are still looking into the keto diet and are considering whether it is the right diet for them to take up. You have the chance to learn about how keto meal prepping and planning works and how convenient it makes the dieting process for you.

Moreover, with all the benefits listed above, you will save time and money while still leading a healthy lifestyle and not compromising on your profession. In fact, you will have more time for your work and a healthy body to see you through the rigors of work.

For those on the keto diet and are not meal prepping and planning, this is another layer to the benefits you are already enjoying from the diet.

1.5 An Overview of Steps to Get Ready for Keto Meal Prepping

Now that you know the benefits of a keto meal prep plan, we will have an overview of the steps and what you need to get ready for meal prepping. As much as there may be nuances in prepping the different meals, the general structure of getting ready for food prepping will remain the same throughout.

Here is what you need to do:

- **Step 1: Decide what to eat.**

  Pick a day of the week when you have enough time to outline a meal plan for the whole week.

  Decide your meals by doing the following:

    - Evaluate what you want to eat each day of the coming week for breakfast, lunch, and supper. Include snacks or desserts as you may want.
    - Slot your picks in a calendar to correspond to the days and mealtimes.
    - Go for ready recipes that have calories indicated and, if possible, macros listed so that you can easily adapt them to your preferences.
    - Account for the number of people who will be served.
    - Make it simple, having one meal more than once, either cooked or as a leftover.
    - Print or write down the recipe for each meal and the ingredients as required.

- **Step 2: Map and plan the meals you have chosen.**

  The next thing after picking out the meals you want for a week is to map out and plan the meals to meet keto nutritional requirements. Create different nutrition combinations for fat, carbohydrates, proteins, and vegetables. These combinations will help you with portioning the meals and drawing a supporting list of things to shop for.

- **Step 3: Make a shopping list, pick a shopping day, and shop for the ingredients.**

    Write down the ingredients and other requirements, pick a convenient day to buy the items on your shopping list, and then shop for the items.

- **Step 4: Cook the keto meals.**

    This is the final step in the prepping process. Once you have the ingredients ready, it is time to prep the meals and cook them accordingly.

Quick Start Action Step

For your meal prepping, follow the four steps above to cover all bases. Decide the keto diet meals you want and get the recipes, map and plan the individual meals, do a detailed shopping list and buy the required ingredients, and finally prep the ingredients and cook the meals.

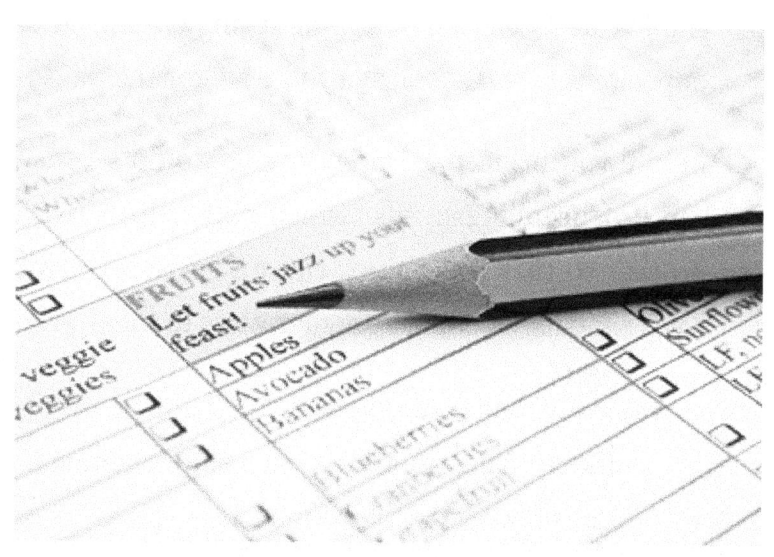

Chapter 2: How to Begin Meal Prepping

In this chapter, we shall look at the things you need to have ready to begin meal prepping. We shall discuss the must-have kitchen equipment for meal prepping. We shall also look at how to stock your pantry with keto essentials and the type of storage containers you need for storing the meals you prepare.

2.1 Getting Ready for Keto Meal Prepping

When you have everything in place for meal prepping—the basic kitchen utensils and equipment, the meal prepping ingredients, and storage containers—you make meal prepping much easier. Preparing the pantry staples and kitchen equipment may seem time-consuming, but the opposite is true. It will save you time for the days and weeks to come.

Before you begin meal prepping, it would be wise to know the different ways of prepping meals, which will help with saving you time on the process so that you do not end up spending a whole day prepping your week's meals. The most popular ways to meal-prep include the following:

- Individual portions: Cooking fresh meals and portioning them into individual grab-and-go meals. Refrigerate and eat over the next few days. This is best for lunches.
- Ready-to-cook meals: This involves prepping ingredients for different meals in advance to save time when cooking.
- Cooking full meals in advance: You cook all the meals you want and refrigerate them. Warm them at mealtimes. This is convenient for dinners.
- Batch cooking: Cooking a large portion of one recipe and then dividing it into several portions, freezing them, and eating them for weeks or months. Best for lunches and dinners.

The method you choose for prepping your meals will be your preference and will probably be determined by your schedule and time management goals. Mixing different meal-prepping methods can also work depending on your unique circumstances.

2.2 The Benefits of Having Essentials Ready for Meal Prepping

Meal prepping can be challenging if you are a beginner, and you should, therefore, not be surprised nor discouraged. It is very easy to get caught up in the nitty gritty in trying to get it right. However, once you have the basics learned, you should take it easy and be practical. Do not try to do everything at once, and do not seek perfection. You should allow yourself room to wriggle and make mistakes from which you will learn from as time goes by.

Prepping meals is important for getting the keto diet right. Planning and prepping your meals ahead of time will help you stay within the recommended portions and nutritional counts.

Additionally, having the essentials of meal prepping ready—the equipment, ingredients, containers, and other requirements—may save you time in prepping and cooking. You will be stress-free and will get more done faster if you have things ready, having your meals for the week ready in no time and leaving the rest of the day to rest.

2.3 The Essentials and Requirements for Meal Prepping

There are a number of kitchen equipment and tools that you must have to begin meal prepping. Additionally, you must have the essential ingredients for your recipes ready, as well as certain must-have keto diet ingredients. Having these kitchen tools and keto pantry staples is a time-saver.

The lists below have the essentials you should have ready for successful and stress-free meal prepping:

Kitchen Equipment and Tools

The following are some of the basic kitchen equipment and tools you need for prepping your keto-friendly meals. There are many household stores where you can get what you want at very affordable prices, as well as bargain sites like Amazon.

a. Skillet

A cast iron skillet is a must-have in your kitchen for easy meal prepping, and it lasts a long time. It is easy to clean and offers better service than a pan. These are easy to clean and safer than using a cheap Teflon-covered pan. Plus, it helps keep your iron levels up.

b. Chef's knife

Since you will be doing a lot of dicing and slicing, you need a dependable knife that will serve you well for a long time. Getting a high-quality chef's knife will make cutting and slicing very easy.

c. Blender or food processor

The keto diet is full of meals and recipes that will require a blender or food processor. Certainly, for keto smoothies, salad dressings, homemade nut butter, etc., you will need one. A blender and processor in one is a good option instead of having two.

d. Instant Pot or pressure cooker or slow cooker

This is the perfect kitchen essential for slow and long cooking. Some of the keto recipes you will encounter will need you to cook broths and soups or slow cook meats, which require you to have a slow cooker. You will have other parts of a recipe slow cooking as you prep others.

e. Nonstick baking paper

Your keto oven meals and bakes will require nonstick oven paper.

f. Kitchen scale

You will need a kitchen scale to weigh some foods and ingredients. This is a perfect product for keto diet meal prep beginners who are just learning how to stay in ketosis.

There are so many kitchen tools that you can have to make your work easier in the kitchen. Here, we have only listed what we think are the essentials for you to have for keto meal prepping.

Stocking the Pantry with the Essentials

For the pantry, there are general cooking ingredients that you must have, and then there are keto essential ingredients that you will need to stock so that you do not miss a recipe item or make several time-wasting trips to the shop.

The following are what you should have for keto meal prepping:

1. Almond flour
2. Avocado oil
3. baking powder and baking soda
4. Butter (preferably grass-fed)
5. Celery salt
6. Cheese(s)
7. Cream cheese
8. Cinnamon
9. Cocoa powder
10. Coconut aminos
11. Coconut flour
12. Coconut oil
13. Eggs (free range and pastured recommended)
14. full-fat coconut milk
15. Garlic cloves
16. Garlic powder
17. Ground beef (grass-fed recommended)
18. Heavy cream
19. Hot sauce
20. Keto sweeteners (erythritol, monk fruit, stevia, Swerve, Truvia)
21. Mayonnaise

22. MCT oil powder
23. Mustard (Dijon or yellow)
24. Nuts and seeds
25. Nut butters
26. Olive oil
27. Oregano
28. Parsley
29. Pumpkin pie spice
30. Red pepper flakes
31. Red wine vinegar
32. Sugar-free spices
33. Salt and pepper
34. Sour cream
35. Thyme
36. Unsweetened yogurt
37. Vanilla extract
38. high-fat oils

These are simply the essentials. You may stock as many as you want as long as they fit in the keto diet.

2.4 Storage Containers to Use

The containers you choose for storing your food storage can turn your food from a fabulous meal to an unenjoyable dish. Glass containers are the best for food storage because they are safe for microwave heating and warming. They do not have harmful chemicals as found in plastics.

In fact, use only glass containers for keto meal prepping, and make sure they are made for the microwave and oven.

Recommended Food Storage Container Specifications

- Airtight—to keep food fresh.

- BPA-free microwavable containers—go for Pyrex glassware.
- Compartmentalized containers—to enable you to have the different parts of a meal in one container.
- Freezer-safe containers—to limit freezer burn.
- Leak-proof
- Stackable—for better space management.

There are a lot of container options on the market for you to pick from. As long as they can be used in the oven or the microwave to heat or warm your food and they meet the recommended food storage specifications above, the glass container will be good for use. You should also get them in different sizes so that you can pack different portions and recipes conveniently.

A high-quality food storage container should ensure that the nutrients in the food do not deteriorate quickly and that the food stays fresh and retains its taste.

Quick Start Action Step

Now that you know the basics required of you to have before meal prepping, if you are a beginner, we would recommend shopping for the items you do not have a day before the actual meal prep, preferably when you will be shopping for recipe ingredients.

Meal planning and prepping is best on weekends, when you are likely to have sufficient time to do it without distractions and disruptions. Saturday for shopping and Sunday for prepping works well.

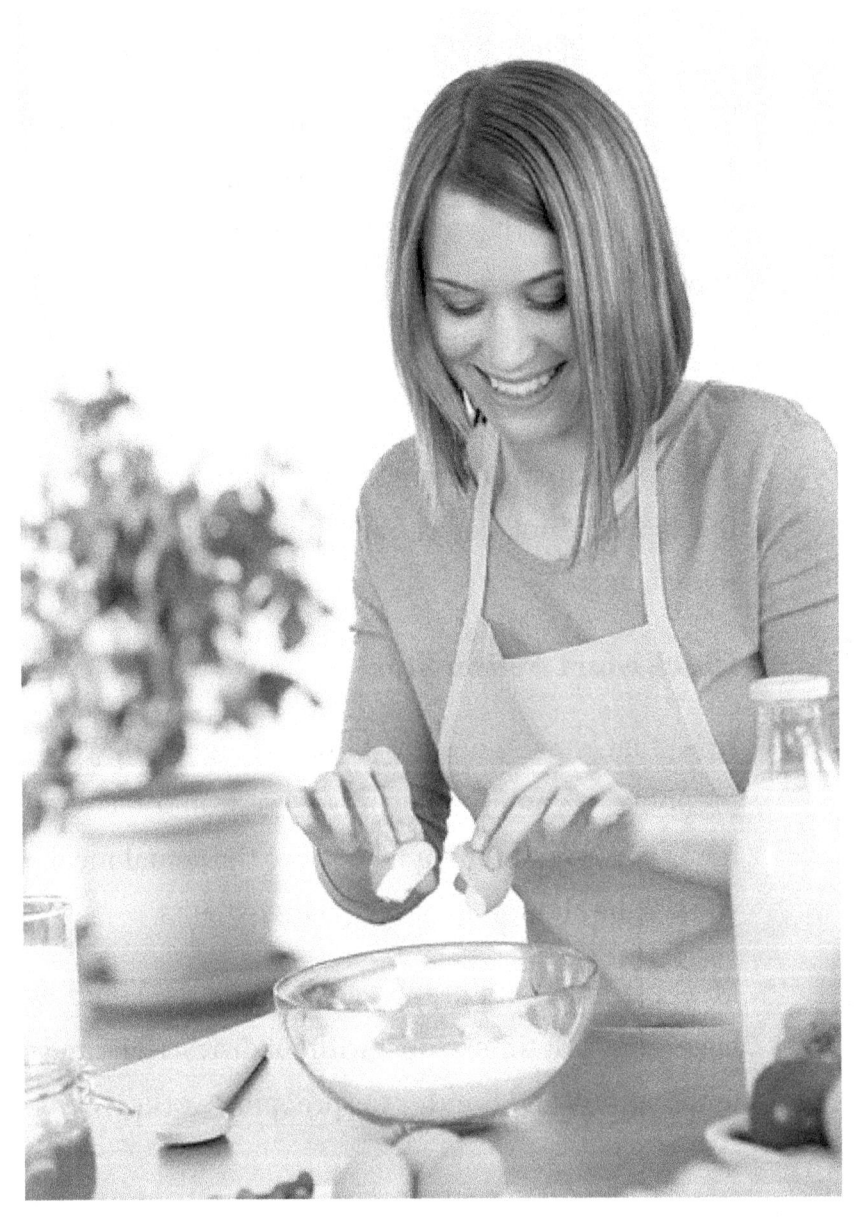

Chapter 3: Easy Steps to Meal Prepping

This chapter will outline easy steps to guide you through successful keto meal prepping from beginning to end. You will mention the benefits of going by these steps and discuss each step of keto meal prepping in detail. Additionally, we will give you insights on how to calculate macros and why that is important.

3.1 How to Calculate Macros

We already know that for you to be successful with ketogenic dieting, you must plan every step and ensure that everything is done right. Calculating macros is one of the important aspects of ensuring success if you are on a keto diet.

To eat right, you need to pick the right keto recipes, which will require you to look at the calorie and macro contents of each meal and each day. Macros are the three main macronutrients of the keto diet, namely, fat, protein, and carbohydrates. While a regular diet is heavily reliant on carbs, the keto diet is fat-oriented.

You will need to eat foods with high quantities of fat, moderate protein, and very little carbs. It is easy when said; however, getting it right with every meal needs a keen tracking of the macro content. Every meal you eat on keto meal plan should be 75% fat, 20% protein, and 5% total carbohydrates.

For instance, if you are on 2,000 calories per day, the breakdown will be as follows:

- 1,500 calories or 167 grams of fat

- 400 calories or 100 grams of protein

- 100 calories or 25 grams of carbs

To achieve and maintain ketosis, you will have to make sure that your nutrients per meal are maintained at the quantities broken down above and have carbs at 25 grams or below.

For beginners, making macro calculation is a must. The good news is that the longer you stay on the diet, the easier it will get, and you will easily know your ratios depending on the recipe once you are familiar with the meals.

To calculate macros effectively, you will need a ketogenic calculator which will give you calculations for a classic ketogenic diet (75% fat, 20% protein, 5% carbohydrate), which is the recommended keto diet and a specialized macro calculation function for more specificity in calculation of macros where you can input specific figures for fat, protein, and carbohydrate.

How to Use the Ketogenic Macro Calculator

Here is how the calculator works:

- **Step 1: Pick the macro calculating option—standard or specialized.**

    You pick between the standard ketogenic diet calculator and the specialized macronutrient calculator. Beginners and those on the classic keto diet should work with the standard option, which is straightforward and is easy to use. It works on the basis of the standard percentages of carbs, fats, and protein in the normal keto diet.

The second option, specialized macro calculator, computes specific carb and protein targets, which you choose, thus not based on the classic keto ratios. There are several reasons why some people would want to do this.

It is important to note that this function is best left to those who have been on keto for some time, have achieved ketosis, and have a good understanding of how the diet works for them and interacts with their bodies.

When to use the standard keto calculation option:

- If you do not know your ketosis macros ratios.

- If you want exact ratios for every meal.

- If you are new to the ketogenic diet.

- If your reason for dieting is simply to lose, gain, or maintain weight.

When to use the specialized macronutrient calculation option:

- Pregnant or breastfeeding women who are measuring macros based on doctor advice.

- If you are adjusting macros ratios because of the keto rash.

- If your doctor recommends different macros ratios from the standard.

- If you know the exact grams of carbs and protein macros to aim for.

- If you have specific macro needs, e.g., an athlete.

- If you are on a high-protein keto diet.

The specialized macronutrient calculator should be used by those on keto who have special macros needs because of issues, like a very active lifestyle (athlete), a medical condition, or pregnancy.

- **Step 2: Enter the basal metabolic rate (BMR) details.**

The next step is to add your basic details. The calculator needs information about your age, gender, height, and weight to come up with your basal metabolic rate (BMR)—the amount of energy your body spends, per unit, while at rest.

How your bio details affect Your BMR:

- Age: BMR shrinks with age, starting after about thirty years, because of muscle mass decline.

- Gender: The body composition and performance of female and male differ.

- Height and weight: Needed to compute your unique body composition.

- **Step 3: Input how active you are.**

Next, the calculator needs to factor in how active you are. Physical activity level (PAL) determines how much energy you burn daily when active. Your BMR outcome and PAL will be combined to calculate your total daily energy expenditure (TDEE)—the number of calories your body burns daily. This will then decide the daily calorie content to compensate what you burn.

- **Step 4: Set dieting goals.**

This is the point when you tell the calculator why you are on the keto diet. What results are you working toward? You state whether you want to maintain, gain, or lose weight, inputting a calorie deficit, surplus, or a zero depending on what you want to achieve.

For example:

Choosing 20% calories deficit reduces your daily calories by 20% of what you actually need, thus resulting in moderate weight loss.

- **Step 5: Use the specialized calculator's advanced fields—body fat percentage, protein ratio, and total carb intake.**

This is the step in the specialized calculator option that factors in specific macro ratios as entered. The body fat percentage, protein ratio, and carbs intake are considered. *Body fat percentage*, which determines lean body mass, enables calculation of a more accurate TDEE. Subsequently, the protein ratio you require per day for weight loss without losing muscle is arrived at.

3.2 The Benefits of Following These Steps for Keto Goals

The benefits of keto meal prep planning are probably what has got you interested in the keto diet in the first place or what led you to pick this book. The benefits of the steps here are the overall keto meal prepping and planning benefits as discussed in detail earlier in chapter 1. Here is a quick recap of the advantages following these steps for meal prepping before we discuss the steps in detail.

The following is a list of the benefits of keto meal prep planning:

1. It saves time as compared to cooking daily.

2. Meal prepping is cheaper than cooking every day.

3. You do not decide what to eat every day.

4. You have better control your food portions.

5. You have better calorie and macro management.

6. Homemade food, especially by yourself, is delicious, healthier, and safer.

7. You have everything ready for cooking ahead of time.

3.3 Keto Meal Prep Planning Steps

1. *Plan the Meal Prep*

Planning entails picking a day for keto meal prepping, picking the meals you want for the week, and settling on the right recipes for the meals.

- *Pick the prepping day.*

    The first thing to do is to pick the day for prepping the meals. Sunday is the best day because most people are off work and can enlist the help of others if you want. Some people opt for two days in a week to prep, which allows them to split meal prepping into two, usually Sunday and Wednesday.

- *Choose the meals.*

    Once you have a day or have decided to split meal prepping into two days, choose the meals you want. Since we are focused on planning for a whole week, choose all the meals, desserts, and snack that you want. Ensure that the meals are healthy and are keto compliant. You can also mark the meals on a calendar at this point.

- *Pick meal recipes.*

    Once you know the meals you want, the next thing to do is to find keto recipes for the meals you have chosen. Keep the calories and macros in mind when picking the recipes so that you balance the meals correctly.

    Beginners should choose easy recipes with a few ingredients. Even better, go for recipes that have similar ingredients—for instance, different meals with meats or vegetables—to make shopping and cooking easier.

Knowledge of how macronutrients are converted into calories will help you keep the right ratios. When choosing recipes, select the ones that you want to eat and will enjoy. It should not just be healthy, you should be happy about it.

- *Write down the week's keto menu.*

Once you have the recipes, write them down in the order you want to eat them during the week. Write down or print out the recipes so that you have them to follow on prep day. It also helps to craft the order in which the food is prepared. Start with the more engaging meals and finish up with the easy ones, like those for breakfast, desserts, and snacks.

- *Pick a prep day.*

This is the point where you decide if you want to do it on Saturday or Sunday or if you want to prep twice, say on Wednesday and Sunday. As advised earlier, it works best to prep a day after shopping, or you can choose to prep the same day you shop.

2. Write Down the Shopping List

Draw a shopping list of the ingredients from each of the recipes you have settled on. Break down the list into food categories—dairy, meat, vegetables, etc. The list must have the exact quantities of each ingredient as per the keto recipes. Avoid packaged and processed products.

Tip: Always check your fridge, freezer, and pantry to confirm what you have so that you do not overstock.

3. Go Shopping for the Items You Listed

Once you have the shopping list, all you have left is to buy what you need before you embark on the actual prepping. As said earlier, pick a convenient shopping day and time so that you are not drained by the experience. Shop when there is less traffic in the shops so that you will easily get what you want to leave.

Apart from the recipe items, buy the keto pantry essentials we listed earlier—any kitchen equipment and storage containers enough for the meals you will be preparing. Make sure you have your shopping list and stick to buying the items in it as planned.

4. Cook and Store the Meals

This is the point you have been preparing for—making the effort count and turning the recipes into delicious meals. Have all ingredients ready and the recipes out when doing this and follow them step by step.

Cooking can be tricky and may take longer than planned or suggested by the respective recipes, but keep going. It will be easier as you go along. Read through the recipes to understand what you need to do and how to do it. It is a good idea to start with those meals with the longest preparation process.

Those that need to be marinated or simmered for long periods should be dealt with first before the cooking day or hour so that everything is ready for the finalization of the dishes. All the veggies and meats that need to be prepared (cutting, slicing, dicing, marinating, etc.) should be done earlier so that they are ready on your cooking day. You may want to do this on shopping day after making your purchases or very early in the morning on prep day.

When packing the foods for storage, take into account the storage life of the various constituents of the meals packed, as well as recommended refrigeration times after cooking. For example, cut vegetables, like onions and peppers, will stay fresh under refrigeration for up to three days. Leafy vegetable if dried will last about a week, and cooked grains and meat dishes should be eaten within four days of cooking. Warm the meals at respective healthy temperatures when eating.

Tips:

- Newbies to keto and to meal prep should begin small and gradually prepare more meals once they learn and identify their favorite recipes and get a handle on meal prepping respectively.

- When you start, choose simple recipes with a few ingredients and pick recipes with similar ingredients to shorten your shopping list and make cooking faster.

- If you are a beginner, you do not have to do a whole week. Try preparing three meals for starters to have a feel of the process.

- Start with some recipes that you have prepared before.

- Plan meals around seasonal produce for freshness and price value.

- Preparing the same dish for two or three mealtimes is a good energy-saving and time-saving idea for beginners.

Quick Start Action Step

Meal prepping is not a complicated process, is it? It may seem like at first, especially for a beginner when you move from reading to actual doing.

Now what you need to do is to act on the steps learned here and follow through on the keto meal prep planning. Pick the meals you want and decide the meal prep day. Draw your shopping list to cover the ingredients, buy everything you need, and finally cook your meals and store them for the week ahead.

There is no better satisfaction than eating a delicious healthy meal prepared by yourself.

Chapter 4: Simple Go-To Recipes to Start

Meal prepping is not as it seems for beginners. In fact, it can be overwhelming since you have to pick out recipes fit for a diet that you have just started following, then prepare several meals on this new dieting regime. Find here simple, easy-to-fix go-to recipes to make on a weekend that you can start with.

Some of the benefits of using the recipes shared here for beginners:

- Time-saving
- Easy to prepare and short cooking times
- Ketogenic compliant
- Avoid the stress of identifying meals
- Money-saving

4.1 The Recipes

Here are simple keto recipes for beginners:

Breakfast Recipes

1. Bacon-and-Egg Muffins (Cups)

Bacon-and-eggs muffins are a quick low-carb breakfast fix for breakfast and will give your body an infusion of energy and protein. It is high in fat, which is perfect for the keto diet. Once you have everything baking in the oven, you can work on with other things as you wait for the oven ringer. Use gluten- and nitrate-free bacon.

Prep: 5 minutes

Cook: 35 minutes

Total: 40 minutes

Calories (350), fat (26 g), carbs (1 g), protein (26 g)

Ingredients

- 12 slices sugar-free bacon
- 8 eggs
- 1/2 cup shredded cheddar cheese
- a pinch of salt
- 1/4 teaspoon black pepper
- 1/4 cup diced green onions/scallions
- 1/2 cup chopped fresh spinach

Instructions

1. Preheat oven to 350°F.
2. Put the cheese, eggs, pepper, and salt together and whip with a fork.

3. Prepare 12 muffin tins. Spray them with nonstick cooking oil.

4. Place the bacon strips inside each muffin cup on the sides.

5. Fill each muffin cup with the cheese, eggs, pepper, and salt mixture, 3/4 full, ensuring that it is surrounded by the bacon strip.

6. Sprinkle scallions on top of the mixture in the muffin cup.

7. Bake until the egg cups are golden brown, 30–35 minutes.

8. Once baked, scoop them out of the tins with a knife.

9. Serve.

Tip

If prepping the muffins ahead of time, let it cool for 10 minutes after baking, wrap each in saran wrap, and then freeze in a freezer Ziploc. Thaw overnight in fridge and microwave for up to 1 minute to eat.

2. Fried Eggs and Avocado

Prep: 5 minutes

Cook: 8 minutes

Total: 13 minutes

Fat (24.1 g), carbs (12.4 g), protein (13 g)

Ingredients

- 2 eggs

- 1/2 avocado (peeled, pitted, and cubed)

- 1 tablespoon butter

- salt and pepper to taste

Instructions

1. Heat skillet on medium-high heat.

2. Melt butter in skillet.

3. Place eggs into the skillet on one side and place avocado pieces on the other.

4. Stir avocados.

5. Flip eggs after four minutes.

6. Continue to cook eggs for another four minutes.

7. Once eggs are cooked, place them on a plate.

8. Scoop avocado over eggs, and season with salt and pepper if desired.

3. Sausage Patty Avocado Cheese Sandwich

Prep: 5 minutes

Total time: 5 minutes

Protein (22 g), fat (54 g), carbs (7 g)

Ingredients

- 2 sausage patties
- 1 egg
- 1 tablespoon cream cheese
- 1 teaspoon sharp cheddar
- sliced medium avocado
- 1/4–1/2 teaspoon sriracha (to taste)
- salt and pepper to taste

Instructions

- Fry sausages in a skillet over medium heat.

- Melt cream cheese and sharp cheddar in a small bowl.

- Mix cheese and sriracha.

- Season eggs and do an omelet.

- Fill the omelet with cheese and sriracha mixture.

- Complete sandwich.

Snack and Side Recipes

1. Sheet Pan Garlic Parmesan Roasted Broccoli and Green Beans

Prep: 5 minutes

Cook: 20 minutes

Total time: 25 minutes

Ingredients

- 2 heads of broccoli

- broccoli stems, cut into pieces

- 350 grams green beans

- 1 cup grape or cherry tomatoes

- 1/3 cup freshly grated Parmesan cheese

- 1/4 cup olive oil

- half a lemon's juice

- 1 tablespoon minced garlic

- salt and pepper

Instructions

- Preheat the oven to 200°C (400°F).

- Spray nonstick oil on baking sheet or tray.

- Place broccoli and green beans tray.

- Sprinkle Parmesan cheese.

- Sprinkle olive oil and lemon juice.

- Add minced garlic and salt and pepper to season.

- Mix until all the vegetables are covered in dressing.

- Place in oven and bake for 20 minutes.

- Remove sheet and add the tomatoes to the pan after 20 minutes.

- Flip vegetables and put back in the oven to cook evenly.

- Bake for another 5–20 minutes until cooked through. The broccoli florets should be crisp.

- Top with the remaining Parmesan cheese.

2. Kale Chips

Calories (98), fat (7 g), saturated fat (1 g), carbs (6 g), fiber (1 g), protein (3 g)

Ingredients

- 2 large stalks kale

- 1 tablespoon avocado oil

- 1 1/2 tablespoon TBS nutritional yeast

- 1/2 teaspoon garlic powder

- 1/4 teaspoon cumin

- 1/4 teaspoon chili powder

- 1/8 teaspoon cayenne
- 1/4 teaspoon pink salt

Instructions

- Preheat oven to 300°F.
- Oil a large baking sheet.
- Separate kale leaves from the stalk.
- Dry the kale leaves.
- Place the kale leaves in a bowl and sprinkle with 1/2 tablespoon avocado oil.
- Massage oil into the kale leaves with your fingers.
- Sprinkle 1 tablespoon nutritional yeast.
- Add 1/2 tablespoon of yeast.
- Set the leaves to the oiled baking sheet and sprinkle remaining nutritional yeast.
- Bake kale at 300°F for 7–9 minutes
- Watching closely for the right crispy texture.

3. Paleo Scotch Eggs

Prep: 10 minutes

Cook: 30 minutes

Total: 40 minutes

Calories (169), fat (8.2 g), carbohydrates (0.67 g), sugars (0.49 g), protein (23.1 g)

Ingredients

- eggs
- 500 grams (1 pound) minced pork or another meat
- 2 teaspoon herb or spice
- 1/2 teaspoon salt

Instructions

- Boil eggs for 4 minutes.
- Remove eggs and dip in cold water.
- Peel the eggs and dry with paper towel.
- Mix the minced meat with spices.
- Flatten a handful of minced meat like a patty.
- Place the egg patty and cover the egg with the meat.
- Place on an oiled baking tray.
- Bake for 30 minutes at 180°C (350°F).

Lunch Recipes

1. Mexican Turkey Burgers

Prep: 15 minutes

Cook: 15 minutes

Carbs (0.3 g), fat (34.5 g), protein (16.8 g), calories (380)

Ingredients

- 1 pound ground turkey

- 1/3 cup finely chopped red bell pepper

- finely chopped cilantro-1/4 cup

- finely sliced green onions-2

- 2 cloves grated or finely minced garlic

- 1/2 lime, 1 tablespoon juice

- 1/2 teaspoon salt

- 1 tablespoon olive oil

Instructions

- Preheat grill medium to high heat.

- Mix ground turkey, red bell pepper, cilantro, green onions, garlic, lime juice, and salt in a bowl.

- Mix it with a fork.

- Flatten into 4 patties.

- Sprinkle the patties with olive oil and salt.

- Grill the burger patties for 5–8 minutes each side until internal temperature is 165 °F.

2. Cheeseburger Lettuce Wraps

Prep: 15 minutes

Cook: 8 minutes

Carbs (0.3 g), fat (34.5 g), protein (16.8 g), calories (380)

Ingredients

- 2 pounds lean ground beef

- ½ teaspoon seasoned salt

- 1 teaspoon black pepper

- 1 teaspoon dried oregano

- 6 slices American cheese

- 2 large heads iceberg or romaine lettuce, rinsed and dry

- 2 thinly sliced tomatoes

- thinly sliced small red onion

Spread:

- 1/4 cup light mayo

- 3 tablespoons ketchup

- 1 tablespoon dill pickle relish

- salt and pepper

Instructions

- On medium, heat a grill or skillet.

- Mix ground beef, seasoned salt, pepper, and oregano in a large bowl.

- Divide into 6 then roll into balls.

- Flatten each ball into a patty.

- Grill patties for about 4 minutes on each side or until cooked.

- Add cheese to each cooked patty.

- Place each patty on a large piece of lettuce.

- Smear spread.

- Wrap patties with lettuce.

3. *Avocado Tuna Salad Recipe*

Calories (304), fat (20 g), carbohydrates (9 g), protein (22 g)

Ingredients

- 15 ounces (3 small cans) tuna in oil, drained and flaked

- 1 English cucumber, sliced

- 2 large medium avocados (peeled, pitted, and sliced)

- 1 small/medium red onion, thinly sliced

- 1/4 cup cilantro

- 2 tablespoons lemon juice freshly squeezed

- 2 tablespoons extra-virgin olive oil

- 1 teaspoon sea salt to taste

- 1/8 teaspoon black pepper

Instructions

- Mix sliced cucumber, sliced avocado, thinly sliced red onion, drained tuna, and 1/4 cup cilantro in a large bowl.

- Sprinkle the mixture with 2 tablespoons of lemon juice, 2 tablespoons of olive oil, 1 teaspoon of salt, and 1/8 teaspoon black pepper.

Dinner Recipes

1. Spicy Mustard Thyme Chicken and Coconut Roasted Brussels Sprouts

Carbs (0.3 g), fat (34.5 g), protein (16.8 g), calories (380)

Prep: 10 minutes

Cook: 25 minutes

Ingredients

- 1 pound Brussels sprouts, half sliced

- 2 medium chicken breasts, skinless and boneless

- 1/4 cup ground spicy mustard

- 1 tablespoon lemon juice

- 1 teaspoon thyme

- salt and pepper

- 1 tablespoon melted coconut oil

Instructions

- Whisk the spicy mustard, lemon juice, salt, pepper, and thyme.

- Dip chicken breasts and cover with mustard.

- Marinate for 10 minutes in the refrigerator then move to room temperature for 15 minutes before cooking.

- Preheat oven to 350 F.

- Prepare a nonstick oven paper.

- Place Brussels sprouts in a bowl and mix with melted coconut oil, salt, and pepper.

- Place Brussels sprouts on baking sheets.

- Put marinated chicken in a glass baking pan.

- Bake chicken in the oven at 350°F for 10 minutes.

- After 10 minutes, put the Brussels sprouts in the oven and bake both for 15 minutes.

2. Fathead Pizza

Calories: 110 kcal

Prep: 10 minutes

Cook: 10 minutes

Total: 20 minutes

Carbs (0.3 g), fat (34.5 g), protein (16.8 g), calories (380)

Ingredients

- 1 1/2 cups shredded mozzarella cheese

- 2 tablespoons cubed cream cheese

- 2 beaten eggs

- 1/3 cup coconut flour

Instructions

- Preheat the oven to 425°F (218°C) and then line a baking sheet or pizza pan with baking paper.

- Mix cubed cream cheese and shredded mozzarella in a bowl.

- Warm in a microwave for 90 seconds then stir at 45 seconds. Stir again after the 90 seconds until consistently mixed.

- Mix in the eggs and coconut flour.

- Knead into a dough forms. Microwave dough for 10–15 seconds to soften it if it hardens before it is well mixed.

- Spread the dough on a baking-paper-lined baking pan to about 1/4 or 1/3 inches thick.

- Poke holes with a toothpick or fork on the crust.

- Bake for 6 minutes.

- Poke more holes in any places with bubbles forming.

- Bake for an additional 3–7 more minutes until it turns golden brown.

3. Pan Lemon Chicken with Asparagus

Prep: 5 minutes

Cook: 25 minutes

Total: 30 minutes

Calories (298), fat (11 g), carbohydrates (13 g), protein (35 g)

Pan lemon chicken with braised asparagus in lemon mustard sauce is a healthy meal. It is also easy to prepare and is packed with keto nutrients.

Ingredients

- 4 skinless chicken breasts boneless

- 1/4 cup plain gluten-free flour or tapioca flour for paleo

- 2 tablespoons olive oil

- 3/4 teaspoon sea salt plus more for seasoning

- 1/2 teaspoon ground black pepper

- ground black pepper for seasoning

- 1 pound asparagus stalks, trim and cut in half

- 2 cloves crushed garlic

- 3 tablespoons fresh lemon juice

- zest of 1/2 lemon

- 1 tablespoon Dijon mustard

- 1 cup chicken stock, buy low-sodium stock

- 1 tablespoon fresh parsley, roughly chopped

- parsley for garnishing

Instructions

- Pound the chicken breasts between two plastic cling wraps, evenly thick. It will enable the chicken to cook evenly and make it more tender. If the chicken breasts are too thick, slice them lengthwise in half.

- Coat the breasts in the flour, salt, and pepper in a dish or bowl. Mix well until completely covered.

- Add 1 tablespoon of olive oil in a large skillet and heat on medium-high heat. Add the chicken to the skillet and cook each side for about 5 minutes or until golden brown once the oil is hot. Make sure it is cooked through.

- Remove the chicken and set on a serviette-lined plate once cooked.

- In the remaining 1 tablespoon of olive oil, sauté the asparagus stalks in the skillet for one minute. Add garlic and sauté for another minute until it gives an aroma.

- In a small bowl or cup, whisk together the lemon juice and mustard until fully mixed. Pour into the skillet with the asparagus along with the chicken stock and the zest. Bring the liquid to a boil and then reduce down to a simmer. Cover and let it cook for another 3–4 minutes or until the asparagus is tender.

- Stir in the parsley and then add the chicken back to the pan and rotate the breasts to coat in the liquids. Taste the sauce and season with more salt and pepper as needed.

Desserts Recipes

1. Keto Avocado Brownies

This avocado dessert is delicious and creamy. It is a great keto recipe with low-carb content, and it is made from sugar-free chocolate.

Prep: 10 minutes

Cook: 35 minutes

Total: 45 minutes

Ingredients

- 250 grams avocado (about 2)
- 1/2 teaspoon vanilla
- 4 tablespoons cocoa powder
- 1 teaspoon stevia powder or monk fruit powder
- 3 tablespoons refined coconut oil or butter, ghee, shortening, lard
- 2 eggs
- 100 grams melted Lily's chocolate chips

Dry Ingredients

- 90 grams blanched almond flour
- 1/4 teaspoon baking soda
- 1 teaspoon baking powder
- 1/4 teaspoon salt
- 60 milliliters erythritol (or xylitol)

Instructions

- Preheat the oven to 350°F (180°C).
- Blend the avocado until smooth.
- Add the ingredients one at a time until all are in, but for the dry ingredients, put them in the blender or food processor.
- Mix together the dry ingredients and whisk. Add to the food processor and mix until combined.
- Pour the blended mixture evenly on a baking tray and bake for about 35 minutes.

2. Almond Cookies

Protein (4.8 g), carbs (8.6 g), fat (23.2 g), fiber (3.5 g), calories (247)

Ingredients

- 3 tablespoons almond butter, unsweetened
- 1.5 tablespoons coconut oil
- 1/2 large egg
- 1 teaspoon vanilla extract
- 1/8 teaspoon salt
- 1 packet Stevia
- 1/2 cup unsweetened shredded coconut
- 16 almonds
- 1.5 ounces 85% dark chocolate

Instructions

- Preheat oven to 350°F.
- Mix almond butter, coconut oil, egg, vanilla, sea salt, and sweetener in a bowl until well mixed.
- Add the coconut mix in well.
- Form 8 cookies on a baking-paper-lined baking tray using a tablespoon to pour and form into balls.
- Press two almonds into the top of each cookie.
- Bake them for 10 minutes, then let cool.
- Pour molten chocolate onto the oven tray and press the cookies on the chocolate to coat the cookie base with chocolate.
- Sprinkle the remaining chocolate on top of the cookies.

3. Cheesy Bacon-Stuffed Mini Peppers

Prep: 15 minutes

Cook: 12 minutes

Total: 27 minutes

Calories (87), fat (7 g), carbohydrates (1 g), protein (2 g)

Ingredients

- half sliced mini sweet peppers, membranes and seeds removed
- 4 ounces cream cheese
- 2 tablespoons sliced green onions
- 4 slices cooked and crumbled bacon
- 1/2 teaspoon garlic powder
- 1/2 cup shredded cheddar cheese
- Extra cheese for topping
- 1 teaspoon Worcestershire sauce
- cilantro, chopped (optional)

Instructions

- Preheat oven to 400°F.
- Spray nonstick cooking spray on a cookie sheet or oven tray.
- Mix together the bacon, garlic powder, cheddar, cream cheese, green onions, and Worcestershire sauce until smooth.
- Fill the sliced peppers with the mix, a tablespoon each.
- Put on the baking sheet or oven tray and sprinkle with extra cheese.
- Bake for 10–12 minutes until the cheese melts and the peppers are soft.

Quick Start Action Step

There you have it—fifteen great simple go-to recipes for beginners or anyone who wants a quick-fix keto meal. Pick one of the meals from each section daily to start you on the keto diet if you are a newbie. It will save you time and the stress of researching recipes.

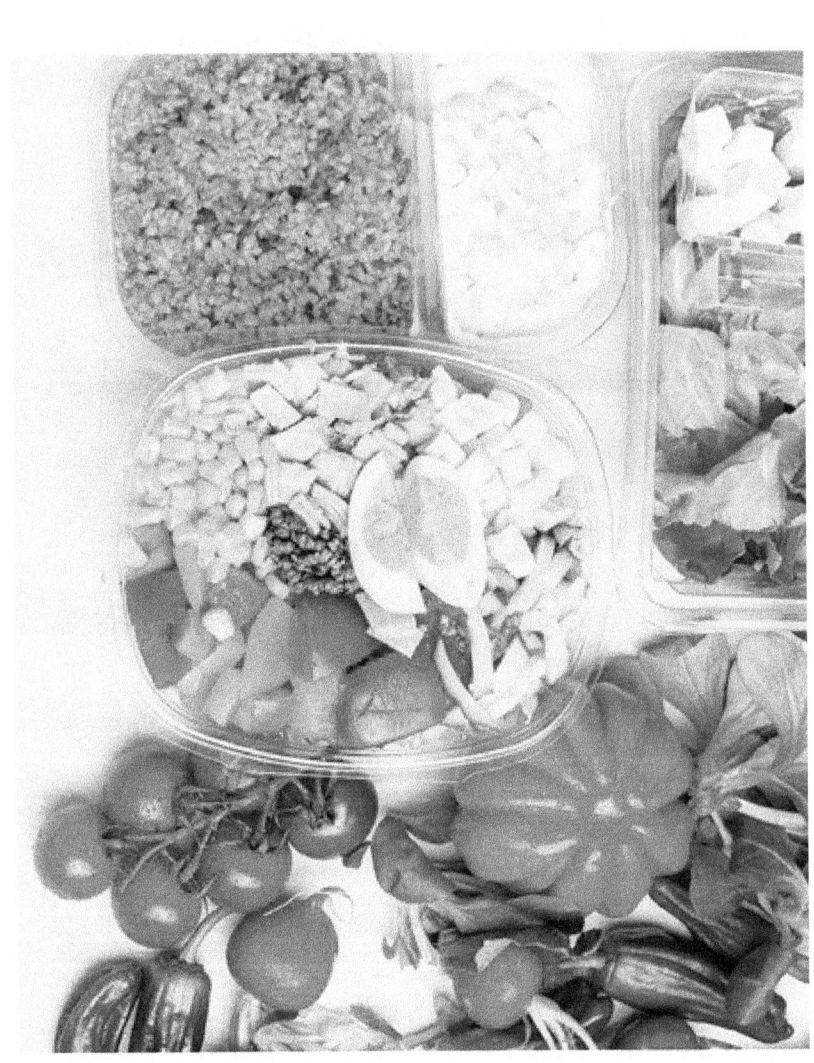

Chapter 5: The Main Recipes

This chapter will outline some of the main keto recipes that you should graduate to once you have a grasp of keto meal prepping from the simple recipes in chapter 4.

5.1 Breakfast Recipes

If you are a beginner on the keto diet, making breakfast may be the most challenging; however, it does not need to be. Preparing a keto breakfast is nothing different from how you prepare other meals. First and most important, start with the macros and then let the macros guide you to the most nutritious foods.

Here is what to do:

- Pick your protein.
- Pair with a low-carb vegetable.
- Include a healthy fat.
- Replace grains with low carb alternatives.
- Remove grains altogether.
- Change the way you make your morning beverage.

1. Ketogenic White Pizza Frittata

These are great when microwaved, reheated in the oven, or just plain cold. This recipe makes use of different cheeses in the frittata base and a top with mozzarella and pepperoni combo. Inside you find spinach that makes sure we get some greens.

The texture is a bit more on the dense side for a frittata due to the melted ricotta and Parmesan cheese inside.

Ingredients

- 12 large eggs
- 9 ounces bag of frozen spinach
- 1 ounce pepperoni
- 5 ounces mozzarella cheese
- 1 teaspoon minced garlic
- 1/2 cup fresh ricotta cheese
- 1/2 cup Parmesan cheese
- 4 tablespoons olive oil
- 1/4 teaspoon nutmeg
- salt and pepper

Instructions

- Place the frozen spinach into the microwave for between 3 and 4 minutes or until defrosted. However, it should not be hot. Squeeze the spinach using your hands and drain as much water as you can. Set it aside.

- Preheat the oven to 375°F. Mix the eggs, olive oil, and spices. Whisk well until properly mixed.

- Add in the ricotta cheese, Parmesan cheese, and spinach. Break the spinach into small pieces using your hands while adding.

- Pour the mixture into a cast iron skillet then sprinkle mozzarella cheese on the top. Add pepperoni on top of that.

- Bake it for half an hour. In case you are using a glass container in place of cast iron, bake it for 45 minutes or until it is completely set.

- Slice it up and devour it. You can top it up using crème fraîche, ranch dressing, or your favorite fatty sauce.

2. Ketogenic Brownie Muffins (6 servings)

Carbs (3.3 g), fat (13.4 g), protein (7 g), calories (183)

These breakfast muffins are rich, hearty, and moist. Far from that, they are low in carbs and high in fibers because of their flaxseed base and wholesome ingredients. Each muffin offers a rich and dark taste of chocolate with a hint of caramel. These muffins are satisfying and can keep you full until lunch hour. Furthermore, they are not hard to make.

Ingredients

- 1 cup golden flaxseed meal
- 1/4 cup cocoa powder
- 1 tablespoon cinnamon
- 1/2 tablespoon baking powder
- 1/2 teaspoon of salt
- 1 large egg
- 2 tablespoons coconut oil
- 1/4 cup sugar-free caramel syrup
- 1/2 cup pumpkin puree
- 1/2 teaspoon vanilla extract

- 1/2 teaspoon apple cider vinegar

- 1/4 cup slivered almonds

Method of Preparation

- Preheat the oven to 350°F and mix all the dry ingredients in a mixing bowl.

- In a different bowl, mix all the wet ingredients.

- Pour all the wet ingredients into the dry ingredients and mix well.

- Line a muffin tin with paper liners and spoon about 1/4 cup of batter into each liner. Sprinkle the slivered almonds over each muffin and gently press for them to stick.

- Bake in the oven for a quarter of an hour.

- Enjoy when warm or cool.

3. Ketogenic Lemon Poppy Seed Muffins (12 servings)

Carbs (1.5 g), fat (11.3 g), protein (3.7 g), calories (129)

They take less time to make and store. They contain 1.5 grams of net carbs per muffin. When fresh, their bottoms crust up well and add the extra crunch when they come out of the oven.

Ingredients

- 3/4 cup blanched almond flour

- 1/4 cup golden flaxseed meal

- 1/3 cup erythritol

- 1 tablespoon baking powder
- 2 tablespoons poppy seeds
- 1/4 cup salted butter, melted
- 1/4 cup heavy cream
- 3 large eggs
- zest of two lemons
- 3 tablespoons lemon juice
- 1 tablespoon vanilla extract
- 25 drops liquid stevia

Method of Preparation

- Preheat the oven to 350 F. In a bowl, use a fork to mix the almond flour, flaxseed meal, erythritol, and poppy seeds.
- Stir in the melted butter, eggs, and the heavy cream until smooth. Make sure that there are no lumps in the batter.
- Once it becomes smooth, add in the baking powder, liquid stevia, vanilla extract, and lemon zest and lemon juice. Mix thoroughly.
- Divide the batter equally among 12 cupcake molds.
- Bake for 20 minutes or until they slightly turn brown.
- Remove from the oven and let it cool for 10 minutes.

4. Bacon Cheddar Chive Omelet (1 serving)

Carbs (1 g), fat (39 g), protein (24 g), calories (463)

The bacon offers a burst of flavor with the eggs and cheese. The chives offer a sweet onion taste.

Ingredients

- 2 slices cooked bacon
- 1 teaspoon bacon fat
- 2 large eggs
- 1 ounce cheddar cheese
- 2 stalks chives
- salt and pepper

Method of Preparation

- Ensure that you have all the ingredients ready because the omelet cooks quite fast. Shred the cheese, precook the bacon, and chop the chives.

- Heat a pan with bacon fat in it at medium-low heat. Add the eggs then season with chives, salt, and pepper.

- As soon as the edges start to set, add the bacon to the center and let it cook for around 30 seconds longer. You then turn off the heat.

- Add the cheese on top the bacon and make sure it's centered. You then take two edges of the omelet and fold them onto the cheese. Hold the edges for a moment as the cheese partially melts to act as an adhesive to hold them in place.

- Do the same with the other edges creating a burrito of sorts. You then flip it over and let it cook for a little longer in the warm pan.

- Serve with extra cheese, bacon, and chives if you like.

5. Ketogenic Breakfast Burger (2 servings)

Carbs (3 g), fat (56 g), protein (30.5 g), calories (655)

This is an option for brunch or heavy breakfast.

Ingredients

- 4 ounces sausage
- 2 ounces pepper jack cheese
- 4 slices bacon
- 2 large eggs
- 1 tablespoon butter
- 1 tablespoon PB fit powder
- salt and pepper

Method of Preparation

1. Begin by cooking the bacon. Lay the strips on a wire rack over a cookie sheet. Bake at 400°F for 25 minutes or until crisp.
2. Mix together butter and PB fit powder in a small container to rehydrate. Set aside.
3. Form sausage patties and cook in a pan over medium to high heat. Turn over when the bottom side is browned.
4. Grate the cheese and have it ready.

5. As soon as the other side of the sausage patty is browned, add the cheese and cover with a lid.

6. Remove the sausage patties with the melted cheese and set aside. Fry an egg in the same pan.

7. Bring everything together—sausage patty, egg, bacon, and the rehydrated PB fit on top.

6. *Chocolate Sea Salt Smoothie*

This smoothie is silky and smooth and tastes great, and it is packed with good fats and ketones.

Benefits of coconut and coconut yogurt:

- Antioxidants
- Vitamins and minerals
- Lactose-free
- High fiber content
- Lauric acid
- Active and live cultures like milk-based yogurts
- Good source of bone-building calcium

Prep: 5 minutes

Cook: 0 minutes

Total time: 5 minutes

Ingredients

- 3 large egg yolks
- 1/3 unsweetened coconut yogurt
- 1 tablespoon tahini

- 1/4 cup cocoa powder
- 20 drops stevia
- 2 scoops Exogenous Ketone Base, chocolate flavored
- 12 ounces water

Instructions

- Mix all the ingredients and blend until smooth.

7. Turkey Sausage Frittata

Frittatas are one of the most loved egg dishes. It combines cheese, cream, meat, sautéed vegetables, and beaten eggs. Frittata is the Italian omelet but cooked a bit differently—beaten eggs mixed with a little liquid, cooked, and then filled with a vegetable, meat, and cheese.

The ingredients are similar to those of the omelet, but it is cooked in a skillet then finished in the oven.

Prep: 10 minutes

Cook: 30 minutes

Calories (240), fat (16.7), carbohydrates (5.5), protein: (16.7)

Ingredients

- 12 ounces ground breakfast sausage, turkey
- 2 bell peppers
- 12 eggs
- 1 cup lactose-free sour cream
- 1 teaspoon pink Himalayan salt
- 1 teaspoon black pepper
- 2 teaspoons butter
- 2 ounces shredded cheddar (optional)

Instructions

- Preheat the oven to 350°F.
- Blend eggs, the sour cream, salt, and pepper on high for 30 seconds.
- Heat a large skillet on medium heat, and once hot, add the butter.
- Slice the bell peppers into strips and throw them into the skillet to sauté until browned and tender for about 6 minutes.
- Remove the bell peppers from the skillet once browned.
- Put the turkey sausage in the skillet and stir while breaking up the meat until it is brown. This should take about eight minutes.
- Flatten the turkey on the bottom of the skillet and add the bell peppers over it evenly.
- Add the egg mix. Pour over everything.
- Place the skillet in the oven and bake for 30 minutes. If you want to add the cheese, sprinkle it over the frittata as soon as you take it out of the oven so it melts.

8. Ketogenic Breakfast Tacos

Prep: 15 minutes

Cook: 10 minutes

Total: 25 minutes

Sugar (2 g), fat (29 g), carbohydrates (4 g), protein (20 g)

Ingredients

- 3 ounces aged cheddar (Tillamook)
- 1 large pastured egg
- 2 slices sugar-free bacon, pastured
- 2 sprigs cilantro
- arugula, a handful

- 1 teaspoon ghee
- a pinch of salt, pepper, and turmeric

Instructions

- Cook bacon. Pan-fry it or pop it in the oven at 350°F until crispy.
- Shred the cheese with a cheese grater.
- Heat skillet on medium-high heat and then add the ghee into the skillet once it is hot.
- Sprinkle the cheese all around into the ghee in the skillet.
- The cheese will start melting almost instantly.
- Once the cheese has melted, crack the egg in the middle of the molten cheese and sprinkle salt, pepper, and turmeric on the yolk.
- Cook for 2 minutes until the egg begins to become opaque and the cheese begins to brown.
- Cook covered for 2 minutes. Seal with a tight-fitting lid and lower the heat.
- Remove. The egg should be fully cooked and the cheese crispy.
- Slide your cheese egg onto a chopping board or dish. Elevate the sides so that the shell cools and hardens and the sides stay up.
- Add the bacon, cilantro, and arugula.

9. Crock-Pot Pumpkin Coconut Breakfast Bars

Prep time: 20 minutes

Serves: 8

Ingredients

- 1 3/4 cup canned pumpkin puree
- 2/3 cup swerve sweetener

- 1 teaspoon raw apple cider vinegar
- 3 eggs, beaten
- 1 cup coconut flour
- 1 tablespoon pumpkin pie spice
- 1/2 tablespoon cinnamon
- 1/2 teaspoon baking soda
- 1/4 teaspoon salt
- 1/3 cup pecan, toasted and chopped

Instructions

1. Line the bottom of the Crock-Pot with parchment paper lightly oiled with cooking oil.
2. In a bowl, mix the pumpkin puree, sweetener, apple cider vinegar, and eggs.
3. In another bowl, mix the coconut flour, pumpkin pie spice, cinnamon, baking soda, and salt.
4. Pour the wet ingredients to the dry ingredients and fold until well mixed.
5. Pour the batter into the Crock-Pot and sprinkle with pecans.
6. Cover with lid. Cook for 3 hours on low or until a toothpick inserted in the middle comes out clean.

Nutrition Information

Calories per serving: 187.4

Carbohydrates: 8.5 g

Protein: 6 g

Fat: 17.2 g

Sugar: 2.5 g

Sodium: 165 mg

Fiber: 3 g

10. Overnight Eggs Benedict Casserole

Prep time: 25 minutes

Serves: 10

Ingredients

- 1 pound Canadian bacon, sliced
- 10 large eggs, beaten
- 1 cup milk
- salt and pepper to taste
- 6 egg yolks
- 2 tablespoons chives, chopped
- 1 1/2 sticks butter, cubed

Instructions

1. Spray cooking oil in the Crock-Pot's ceramic interior.
2. Take the bacon slices at the bottom of the Crock-Pot.

3. In a bowl, mix the eggs and milk. Season with salt and pepper to taste.

4. Pour over the bacon.

5. Close the lid and cook for 1 1/2 hours.

6. Open the lid and take the egg yolks on top. Sprinkle with chopped chives.

7. Continue cooking for another 1 1/2 hours or until the egg mixture is done.

8. While still warm, keep butter on top.

Nutrition Information

Calories per serving: 256

Carbohydrates: 2 g

Protein: 16.2 g

Fat: 21 g

Sugar: 0 g

Sodium: 734 mg

Fiber: 0.3 g

11. Crustless Crock-Pot Spinach Quiche

Prep time: 50 minutes

Serves: 6

Ingredients

- 1 tablespoon ghee

- 2 cups baby bella mushrooms, chopped

- 1 medium red bell peppers, sliced

- 1 package chopped spinach, drained

- 8 eggs, beaten

- 1 cup sour cream

- 1/2 teaspoon salt

- 1/4 teaspoon black pepper

- 1 1/2 cup cheddar cheese, shredded

- 2 tablespoons chives, chopped

- 1/2 cup almond flour

- 1/4 teaspoon baking soda

Instructions

1. Oil the slow cooker with cooking spray.

2. In a skillet, heat the ghee and sauté the mushrooms and bell peppers for 4 hours. Add the kale and cook for another minute. Set aside.

3. In a bowl, mix the eggs and sour cream. Season with salt and pepper. Stir in the cheese and chives. Add the almond flour and baking soda. Mix until well mixed. Stir in the vegetable mixture.

4. Pour the mixture in the Crock-Pot and cook on low for 5 hours or 3 hours on high.

Nutrition Information

Calories per serving: 383.1

Carbohydrates: 7.3 g

Protein: 15.1 g

Fat: 18 g

Sugar: 0 g

Sodium: 547 mg

Fiber: 3.2 g

12. Cheesy and Eggy Breakfast Casserole

Prep time: 35 minutes

Serves: 8

Ingredients

- 12 eggs, beaten
- 3/4 cup half-and-half
- 1/2 teaspoon red pepper flakes
- 1/2 teaspoon salt
- 1/4 teaspoon ground black pepper
- 1 cup cheddar cheese, shredded

- 1 cup Colby cheese, shredded
- 1/2 cup green onions, chopped
- 1 cauliflower head, cut into florets
- 1 pound pork sausages, cooked and sliced
- 1/2 cup red bell peppers, roasted and chopped

Instructions

1. Line the sides of the slow cooker with foil. Oil with cooking spray so that the mixture will not stick on the Crock-Pot.
2. In a mixing bowl, mix the eggs, half-and-half, red pepper flakes, salt, and black pepper. Add the cheeses, onions, and cauliflower florets.
3. Take the sausages at the bottom of the Crock-Pot.
4. Pour over the egg mixture and top with chopped roasted bell peppers.
5. Close the lid and cook for 3 hours or until a toothpick inserted in the middle comes out clean.

Nutrition Information

Calories per serving: 475

Carbohydrates: 5.2 g

Protein: 23 g

Fat: 26.7 g

Sugar: 0.2 g

Sodium: 791 mg

Fiber: 2.1 g

13. Broccoli and Tomatoes Casserole

Prep time: 30 minutes

Serves: 6

Ingredients

- 1 large broccoli, chopped
- 2 tablespoons butter
- Salt and pepper to taste
- 1 1/4 cups cooked bacon, crumbled
- 1 1/2 cups cherry tomatoes, halved
- 2 cups cheddar cheese, shredded
- 8 eggs, beaten
- 1/2 cup whole milk
- 1 bunch scallions, sliced

Instructions

1. Spray cooking spray on the interior of the Crock-Pot.
2. In a mixing bowl, toss the broccoli and butter. Season with salt and pepper to taste.

3. Press the vegetable mixture at the bottom of the Crock-Pot. Add the bacon and tomatoes on top. Add the cheddar cheese.

4. In a mixing bowl, mix the eggs and milk.

5. Pour the egg mixture over the vegetable layers. Sprinkle the scallions.

6. Close the lid and cook on low for 4 hours or until a toothpick inserted in the middle comes out clean.

Nutrition Information

Calories per serving: 486

Carbohydrates: 8.1

Protein: 21.3 g

Fat: 17 g

Sugar: 2.9 g

Sodium: 845 mg

Fiber: 5.4 g

14. Simple Ham-and-Egg Casserole

Prep time: 40 minutes

Serves: 6

Ingredients

- 4 tablespoons butter, melted

- 1/2 green bell pepper, diced

- 1/2 red bell pepper, diced
- 1 small onion, diced
- 1/2 cup ham, diced
- 1/2 cup cheese, shredded
- 6 eggs, beaten
- 1 tablespoon milk
- salt and pepper to taste

Instructions

1. Spray the Crock-Pot with cooking spray.
2. Take melted butter in the Crock-Pot.
3. Add the bell peppers, onions, ham, and cheese in layers.
4. In a mixing bowl, mix the eggs and milk. Season with salt and pepper.
5. Pour over the layers of vegetables and ham.
6. Close the lid and cook for 3 hours on low or until a toothpick inserted in the middle comes out clean.

Nutrition information

Calories per serving: 379.1

Carbohydrates: 7.2 g

Protein: 15 g

Fat: 20.4 g

Sugar: 1.4 g

Sodium: 744 mg

Fiber: 3.9 g

15. *Fluffy Breakfast Omelet*

Prep time: 25 minutes

Serves: 8

Ingredients

- 4 strips bacon, cooked and crumbled
- 1 small onion, chopped
- 2 bell peppers, chopped
- 1 small head broccoli, chopped
- 1/2 cup cheddar cheese, shredded
- 4 egg whites
- 8 eggs, beaten
- 3/4 cup milk
- 2 teaspoons mustard, ground
- 1/2 teaspoon garlic salt
- Salt and pepper to taste

Instructions

1. Oil the Crock-Pot with cooking spray.

2. Arrange in layers the bacon, onion, bell pepper, and broccoli.

3. Top with half of the cheddar cheese.

4. In a mixing bowl, beat the egg whites with a hand mixer until it forms stiff peaks. Set aside.

5. In another bowl, mix the eggs, milk, mustard, and garlic. Season with salt and pepper.

6. Fold the egg-white mixture into the milk mixture gently.

7. Pour over the vegetable mixture.

8. Top with the remaining cheese.

9. Close the lid and cook for 3 hours or until a toothpick inserted in the middle comes out clean.

Nutrition information

Calories per serving: 320

Carbohydrates: 6.5 g

Protein: 22.3 g

Fat: 23.2 g

Sugar: 1.9 g

Sodium: 700 mg

Fiber: 5.3 g

16. Crock-Pot Mediterranean Frittata

Prep time: 30 minutes

Serves: 8

Ingredients

- 8 eggs, beaten
- 1/3 cup milk
- 1 teaspoon dried oregano
- salt and pepper to taste
- 4 cups baby arugula rockets, rinsed and drained
- 1 1/4 cups red peppers, roasted and chopped
- 1/2 cup red onion, sliced thinly
- 3/4 cup goat cheese, crumbled

Instuctions

1. Spray cooking oil inside the Crock-Pot.
2. In a large bowl, mix the eggs, milk, and oregano. Season with salt and pepper.
3. Take the arugula leaves at the bottom of the Crock-Pot. Add the red peppers, onions and goat cheese.
4. Pour over the egg mixture.
5. Cook on low for 3 hours.
6. Serve warm.

Nutrition Information

Calories per serving: 416

Carbohydrates: 7.2 g

Protein: 18.3 g

Fat: 15.9 g

Sugar: 1.3 g

Sodium: 481 mg

Fiber: 4.8 g

17. *Spinach and Mozzarella Frittata*

Prep time: 15 minutes

Serves: 6

Ingredients

- 1 tablespoon extra-virgin olive oil
- 1/2 cup onion, diced
- 3 eggs, beaten
- 1 cup mozzarella cheese, divided
- 2 tablespoons milk
- Salt and pepper to taste
- 3 egg whites, beaten until stiff peaks form
- 1 cup baby spinach, rinsed
- 1 tomato, diced

Instructions

1. In a small skillet, heat oil and sauté the onions for 2 minutes. Set aside.

2. Spray the inside of the Crock-Pot with cooking spray.

3. In a bowl, mix the sautéed onions, eggs, mozzarella cheese, and milk. Season with salt and pepper to taste.

4. Fold the beaten egg whites to the egg mixture. Set aside.

5. Arrange the baby spinach and tomatoes at the bottom of the Crock-Pot.

6. Pour over the egg mixture.

7. Close the lid and cook for 3 hours on low or until a toothpick inserted in the middle comes out clean.

Nutrition Information

Calories per serving: 139

Carbohydrates: 4 g

Protein: 12 g

Fat: 8 g

Sugar: 2 g

Sodium: 435 mg

Fiber: 1 g

18. Artichoke Hearts and Roasted Pepper Frittata

Prep time: 30 minutes

Serves: 8

Ingredients

- 1 can artichoke hearts, drained and cut into small pieces
- 1 cup roasted red peppers, seeds removed and chopped
- 1/4 cup green onions, sliced
- 8 eggs, beaten
- 1/2 cup feta cheese, crumbled
- Salt and pepper to taste
- Chopped parsley for garnish

Instructions

1. Take the artichoke hearts into the oiled Crock-Pot.
2. Add the red peppers and green onions.
3. In a bowl, mix the eggs and cheese. Season with salt and pepper to taste.
4. Pour over the vegetables.
5. Sprinkle parsley on top.
6. Cook on low for 2 1/2 hours.

Nutrition Information

Calories per serving: 322

Carbohydrates: 8.1 g

Protein: 16 g

Fat: 14.2 g

Sugar: 0.6 g

Sodium: 486.2 mg

Fiber: 5.2 g

19. Sausage Cauliflower Breakfast Casserole

Prep time: 40 minutes

Serves: 10

Ingredients

- 1 head cauliflower, chopped finely
- 4 tablespoon unsalted butter, melted
- 2 teaspoons salt
- 1 pound breakfast sausage
- 6 green onions, chopped
- 12 large eggs, beaten
- 1/2 cup mozzarella cheese, shredded

Instructions

1. Take the chopped cauliflower at the bottom of the Crock-Pot. Pour butter and season with salt.
2. Take the sausages and onions on top of the cauliflower bed. Pour over the beaten eggs and top with mozzarella cheese.
3. Cook on low for 3 hours.

Nutrition Information

Calories per serving: 478

Carbohydrates: 5.7 g

Protein: 16.3 g

Fat: 22 g

Sugar: 0.5 g

Sodium: 550 mg

Fiber: 3.8 g

20. Greek Crock-Pot Breakfast Casserole

Prep time: 25 minutes

Serves: 12

Ingredients

- 12 eggs, beaten
- 1/2 cup milk
- 1/2 teaspoon salt
- 1/4 teaspoon black pepper
- 1 teaspoon onion powder
- 1 teaspoon garlic powder
- 1/2 cup sundried tomatoes, soaked overnight
- 1 cup baby bella mushrooms, sliced

- 2 cups spinach
- 1/2 cup feta cheese, shredded

Instructions

1. Lubricate the Crock-Pot with cooking spray.
2. Mix all ingredients in a bowl.
3. Pour the mixture in the Crock-Pot.
4. Cook on low for 4 hours.

Nutrition Information

Calories per serving: 397

Carbohydrates: 7.5 g

Protein: 16.3 g

Fat: 20.3 g

Sugar: 1.2 g

Sodium: 347 mg

Fiber: 3.7 g

21. Coconut Cranberry Quinoa Pudding

Prep time: 40 minutes

Serves: 10

Ingredients

- 3 cups coconut water

- 1 cup quinoa, uncooked
- 1 teaspoon vanilla extract
- 3 teaspoons stevia extract
- 1/3 cup coconut flakes
- 1/3 cup almonds, sliced
- 1/4 cup dried cranberries

Instructions

1. Take all ingredients inside the Crock-Pot.
2. Cook on low for 4 hours.
3. Serve warm.

Nutrition Information

Calories per serving: 246

Carbohydrates: 4 g

Protein: 8 g

Fat: 5 g

Sugar: 3 g

Sodium: 0 mg

Fiber: 5 g

22. *Crock-Pot Breakfast Lettuce Burritos*

Prep time: 30 minutes

Serves: 12

Ingredients

- 12 eggs, beaten
- 1 cup milk
- 1 cup diced ham
- salt and pepper to taste
- lettuce leaves
- cherry tomatoes, halved
- chives, chopped
- sour cream

Instructions

1. Spray the Crock-Pot with cooking spray.
2. In a bowl, mix all ingredients except the lettuce, cherry tomatoes, chives, and sour cream.
3. Cook on low for 4 hours.
4. After an hour, give the egg mixture a stir to create a scrambled-egg-like consistency.
5. Bring together the lettuce burritos by placing the egg mixture on top of the lettuce. Add tomatoes, chives, and sour cream.

Nutrition Information

Calories per serving: 275

Carbohydrates: 4.2 g

Protein: 12.3 g

Fat: 17.7 g

Sugar: 1.2 g

Sodium: 346 mg

Fiber: 2.3 g

23. Breakfast Three-Cheese Shrimps

Prep time: 15 minutes

Serves: 10

Ingredients

- 6 cups chicken stock
- 1 tablespoon garlic powder
- 1 tablespoon onion powder
- 1 teaspoon dried thyme
- salt and pepper to taste
- 1 cup cheddar cheese, shredded
- 4 ounces light cream cheese
- 1/2 cup Parmesan cheese, grated
- 1/2 teaspoon hot sauce
- 2 pounds raw shrimp

- chopped scallions for garnish

Instructions

1. Take all components except the scallions in the slow cooker.
2. Give a stir to incorporate everything.
3. Cook for 30 minutes or an hour on low.
4. Garnish with chopped scallions.

Nutrition Information

Calories per serving: 472

Carbohydrates: 1.2 g

Protein: 17.6 g

Fat: 32 g

Sugar: 0 g

Sodium: 870 mg

Fiber: 0.2 g

Lunch Recipes

1. Broccoli Chicken Zucchini Boats (2 servings)

Carbs (5 g), fat (34 g), protein (30 g)

This is a perfect lunch when you need something a little out of the ordinary. The fillings are perfect and come out with all the flavors.

Ingredients

- 10 ounces zucchini
- 2 tablespoons of butter
- 3 ounces shredded cheddar cheese
- 1 cup broccoli
- 6 ounces shredded rotisserie chicken
- 2 tablespoons sour cream
- 1 stalk green onion
- salt and pepper

Method of Preparation

- Preheat the oven to 400°F and cut the zucchini into halves, lengthwise.
- Using a spoon, scoop out most of the zucchini until you are left with a shell that is about a centimeter thick
- Pour a tablespoon of melted butter into each zucchini boat and season with salt or pepper and place in the oven. This gives the zucchini time to cook as you prepare the filling. This takes about twenty minutes.
- Shred your chicken using two forks so as to pull the meat apart. Measure out 6 ounces and place the rest in the refrigerator for another meal.
- Cut up your broccoli florets until they are bite-sized.
- Mix the chicken and broccoli with sour cream to keep them moist and creamy. Season.

- As soon as the zucchini has cooked, take them out and add the chicken and broccoli filling.

- Sprinkle cheddar cheese on top of your chicken and broccoli and pop them back into the oven for another 15 minutes until the cheese is melted and browning.

- Garnish with chopped green onion.

2. Cheese-Stuffed Bacon-Wrapped Hot Dogs (6 hot dogs)

Carbs (0.3 g), fat (34.5 g), protein (16.8 g), calories (380)

This takes about 10 minutes to prepare.

Ingredients

- 6 hot dogs
- 12 slices of bacon
- 2 ounces cheddar cheese
- 1/2 teaspoon garlic powder
- 1/2 teaspoon onion powder
- salt and pepper

Instructions

- Heat the oven to 400°F. Slit all the hot dogs to create space for cheese.

- Slice 2 ounces cheddar cheese into small and long rectangles. Stuff them into the hotdogs.

- Tightly wrap one slice of bacon around the hotdog

- Go on and tightly wrap the second slice of bacon around the hot dog. Make sure it slightly overlaps with the first slice.

- Poke each side of the bacon and hot dog with a toothpick so as to secure the bacon in place.

- You then set on a wire rack that's on top of a cookie sheet. Season with garlic powder, onion powder, salt, and pepper.

- Bake for between 35 and 40 minutes or until the bacon becomes crispy. You can also broil the bacon on top if needed.

- Serve with some nice creamed spinach.

3. Bacon, Avocado, and Chicken Sandwich (2 servings)

Carbs (2 g), fat (28.3 g), protein (22 g), calories (361)

Ingredients

Keto cloud bread:

- 3 large eggs

- 3 ounces cream cheese

- 1/8 teaspoon cream of tartar

- 1/4 teaspoon salt

- 1/2 teaspoon garlic powder

Filling:

- 1 tablespoon mayonnaise

- 1 teaspoon sriracha
- 2 bacon slices
- 3 ounces chicken
- 2 pepper jack cheese slices
- 2 grape tomatoes
- 1/4 medium avocado

Method of Preparation

- Preheat the oven to 300°F. Start by separating 3 eggs into 2 clean dry bowls.
- Mix the cream of tartar and salt with the egg whites.
- Use an electric mixer to whip the whites until they become soft and foamy.
- In a separate bowl, mix 3 ounces of cubed cream cheese with the egg yolks and beat until they become pale yellow.
- Fold the egg whites into the yolks.
- On a parchment-paper-lined baking sheet, spoon 1/4 cup of the keto cloud bread batter.
- Use a spatula to gently press the tops of the keto cloud bread to form squares. You then sprinkle the tops with garlic powder and bake for about 25 minutes.
- As the keto cloud bread is baking, cook the chicken and bacon with salt and pepper.

- You arrange the sandwich by combining mayo and sriracha and spreading it on the underside of one keto cloud bread. Add the chicken into the mayo mixture.

- Add the two slices of pepper jack cheese and the bacon. Nestle some halved grape tomatoes and spread the mashed avocado on top. Season to taste and top with the other keto cloud bread.

4. Crispy Tofu and Bok Choy Salad (3 servings)

Carbs (5.7 g), fat (35 g), protein (25 g), calories (442)

Tofu that is baked is quite delicious. You get a rich cube that is full of flavor and crunchy on the outsides. Furthermore, raw bok choy is fantastic. It is crunchy and offers a distinct taste to the salad.

Ingredients

Oven baked tofu:

- 15 ounces extra firm tofu
- 1 tablespoon soy sauce
- 1 tablespoon sesame oil
- 1 tablespoon water
- 2 teaspoons minced garlic
- 1 tablespoon rice wine vinegar
- juice made from half a lemon

Bok choy salad:

- 9 ounces bok choy

- 1 stalk of green onion
- 2 tablespoons chopped cilantro
- 3 tablespoons coconut oil
- 2 tablespoons soy sauce
- 1 tablespoon sambal olek
- 1 tablespoon peanut butter
- juice from half a lime
- 7 drops liquid stevia

Instructions

- Begin by pressing the tofu. Place the tofu in a kitchen towel and put something heavy over it. It takes about 4–6 hours to dry out. However, you may need to change the kitchen towel when halfway done.

- After pressing the tofu, work on the marinade. Mix all the ingredients for the marinade. That is soy sauce, sesame oil, water, garlic, vinegar, and lemon.

- Chop the tofu into squares and place them in a plastic bag together with the marinade. Let it marinate for at least half an hour. However, overnight is preferred.

- Preheat the oven to 350°F. Place the tofu on a baking sheet lined with parchment paper. Bake for half an hour.

- When the tofu is cooked, start on the bok choy salad. Chop the cilantro and spring onion.

- You then mix all the other ingredients together apart from lime juice and bok choy. You then add cilantro and the spring onion. You can also microwave the coconut oil for about ten seconds so that it melts.

- When the tofu is almost cooked, add the lime juice into the salad dressing and mix together.

- Chop the bok choy into small pieces.

Remove the tofu from the oven and assemble the salad with tofu, bok choy, and sauce.

5. Avocado Tuna Melt Bites (12 pieces)

Carbs (0.8 g), fat (11.8 g), protein (6.2 g), calories (135)

Their crispy outside combines with the soft creamy filling on the inside.

Ingredients

- 10 ounces canned and drained tuna

- 1/4 cup mayonnaise

- 1 medium avocado, cubed

- 1/4 cup Parmesan cheese

- 1/3 cup almond flour

- 1/2 teaspoon garlic powder

- 1/4 teaspoon onion powder

- salt and pepper

- 1/2 cup coconut oil for frying

Instructions

- Drain a can of tuna and add to a large-sized container where everything will be mixed.

- Add mayonnaise, Parmesan cheese, and spices to the tuna. Mix well.

- Slice the avocado into half and cube it.

- Add avocado into the tuna mixture and fold together. Try not to mash the avocado into the mixture.

- Form the tuna mixture into balls and roll into almond flour, covering them completely. Set aside.

- Heat the coconut oil in a pan over medium heat. As soon as it's hot, add the tuna balls and fry until all sides are crisp.

- Remove from the pan and serve.

6. Portobello Bun Cheeseburgers

Mushrooms, technically, are fungi. However, just like vegetables, portobello mushrooms are packed with essential nutrients and are a great addition to the keto diet.

Unprocessed foods, like mushrooms, help reduce the risk of many health conditions, including obesity, diabetes, and heart disease.

Portobello mushrooms contain two types of dietary fiber (beta-glucans and chitin), which play an important role in weight management. With these dietary fibers, satiety increases and appetite decreases.

Health Benefits of Mushrooms

- Promotes heart health
- Great source of B vitamins
- Boosts immunity
- Low in calories
- Contains disease-fighting antioxidants
- Helps combat inflammation
- Great source of fiber

Prep: 5 minutes

Cook: 15 minutes

Total time: 20 minutes

Calories (336), fat (22.8 g), carbohydrates (5.8 g), carbs (4 g), protein (29.1 g)

Ingredients

- 1 pound grass-fed 80/20 ground beef
- 1 tablespoon Worcestershire sauce
- 1 teaspoon pink Himalayan salt
- 1 teaspoon black pepper
- 1 tablespoon avocado oil
- 6 portobello mushroom caps (destemmed, rinsed, and dabbed dry)
- 6 slices sharp cheddar cheese

Instructions

- Mix ground beef, salt, pepper, and Worcestershire sauce.
- Make the mixture into burger patties.

- Heat avocado oil over medium heat in a large pan and then add portobello mushroom caps.
- Cook for about 3–4 minutes on each side then remove.
- Cook the burger patties in the same pan, 4 minutes on one side and 5 minutes on the other until you get the desired doneness.
- Add cheese to the patties and then cover with a lid to melt the cheese. Do this for about 1 minute.

Garnish Options

- Romaine
- Sugar-free barbecue sauce
- Sliced dill pickles
- Spicy brown mustard

7. Crock-Pot Beef Roast

Prep time: 20 minutes

Serves: 6

Ingredients

- 2 pounds beef chuck roast, trimmed of excess fat
- 1 1/2 teaspoons salt
- 3/4 teaspoon black pepper
- 2 tablespoons fresh basil, chopped
- 1 large yellow onion, chopped
- 4 cloves garlic, minced
- 2 bay leaves

- 2 cups beef stock

Instructions

1. Pat dry the beef roast with a paper towel and rub with salt, pepper, and chopped basil.

2. Take inside the Crock-Pot and spread the onion, garlic, and bay leaves.

3. Pour over the beef stock.

4. Close the lid and cook on low for 10 hours until tender.

Nutrition Information

Calories per serving: 234

Carbohydrates: 2.4 g

Protein: 33.1 g

Fat: 10.3 g

Sugar: 0.9 g

Sodium: 758.2 mg

Fiber: 0.5 g

8. Chipotle Barbecue Chicken

Prep time: 20 minutes

Serves: 5

Ingredients

- 1/4 cup water

- 1 1/4 ounce boneless chicken breasts, skin removed
- 1 1/4 ounce boneless chicken thighs, skin removed
- salt and pepper to taste
- 2 tablespoons chipotle Tabasco sauce
- 1 onion, chopped
- 4 tablespoons unsalted butter
- 1 cup tomato sauce
- 1/3 cup apple cider vinegar
- 1/2 cup water
- 2 tablespoons yellow mustard
- 1/4 teaspoon garlic powder

Instructions

1. Take all ingredients in a Crock-Pot.
2. Give everything a stir so that the chicken is coated with the sauce.
3. Close the lid and cook on low for 8 hours.

Nutrition Information

Calories per serving: 482

Carbohydrates: 3 g

Protein: 29.4 g

Fat: 18.7 g

Sugar: 0 g

Sodium: 462 mg

Fiber: 0.3 g

9. Spicy Shredded Chicken Lettuce Wraps

Prep time: 15 minutes

Serves: 8

Ingredients

- 4 chicken breast, skin and bones removed
- 1 cup tomato salsa
- 1 teaspoon onion powder
- 1 can green chilies, diced
- 1 tablespoon Tabasco sauce
- 2 tablespoons lime juice, freshly squeezed
- salt and pepper to taste
- 2 large heads iceberg lettuce, rinsed

Instructions

1. Take the chicken breast in the Crock-Pot.
2. Pour over the tomato salsa, onion powder, green chilies, Tabasco sauce, and lime juice. Season with salt and pepper to taste.

3. Close the lid and cook for 10 hours.

4. Shred the chicken meat using a fork.

5. Take on top of lettuce leaves.

6. Garnish with sour cream, tomatoes, or avocado slices if needed.

Nutrition Information

Calories per serving: 231

Carbohydrates: 3 g

Protein: 23 g

Fat: 12 g

Sugar: 0.5 g

Sodium: 375 mg

Fiber: 2 g

10. Bacon Cheeseburger Casserole

Prep time: 50 minutes

Serves: 8

Ingredients

- 2 pounds ground beef
- 1/2 onion, sliced thinly
- 1/2 teaspoon salt
- 1/2 teaspoon black pepper

- 1 (15-ounce) can cream of mushroom soup
- 1 (15-ounce) can cheddar cheese soup
- 1/2 pounds bacon, cooked and crumbled
- 2 cups cheddar cheese, grated

Instructions

1. Brown the ground beef and onions in a skillet over medium heat. Season with salt and pepper to taste.
2. Take the beef in the Crock-Pot and add the cream of mushroom soup and cheese soup.
3. Pour in the bacon and half of the cheddar cheese. Give a stir.
4. Cook on low for 4 hours.
5. An hour before the cooking time is over. Add the remaining cheese on top.

Nutrition Information

Calories per serving: 322

Carbohydrates: 2 g

Protein: 36 g

Fat: 21 g

Sugar: 0 g

Sodium: 271 mg

Fiber: 1.3 g

11. Crock-Pot Ranch Chicken

Prep time: 55 minutes

Serves: 6

Ingredients

- 2 pounds boneless chicken breasts
- 3 tablespoons dry ranch dressing mix
- 3 tablespoons butter
- 4 ounces cream cheese

Instructions

1. Take the chicken in the Crock-Pot. Pour the ranch dressing and rub on the chicken.
2. Add the butter and cream cheese.
3. Close the lid and cook for 7 hours on low.
4. Shred the chicken before serving.

Nutrition Information

Calories per serving: 266

Carbohydrates: 0 g

Protein: 33 g

Fat: 12.9 g

Sugar: 0 g

Sodium: 167 mg

Fiber: 0 g

12. Coconut Cilantro Shrimp Curry

Prep time: 40 minutes

Serves: 4

Ingredients

- 1 can light coconut milk
- 15 ounces water
- 1/2 cup Thai red curry sauce
- 2 1/2 teaspoons lemon juice
- 1 teaspoon garlic powder
- 1/4 cup cilantro
- salt and pepper to taste
- 1 pound shrimps, heads removed only

Instructions

1. Take the coconut milk, water, and curry sauce in the Crock-Pot.
2. Stir in the lemon juice, garlic powder, and cilantro. Season with salt and pepper to taste.
3. Cook on high for 23 hours.
4. Add the shrimps and cook on high for 10 minutes.

Nutrition Information

Calories per serving: 211

Carbohydrates: 2 g

Protein: 18.2 g

Fat: 22 g

Sugar: 0 g

Sodium: 135 mg

Fiber: 0.8 g

13. Crock-Pot Butter Masala Chicken

Prep time: 45 minutes

Serves: 8

Ingredients

- 1 tablespoon olive oil
- 9 cloves of garlic, crushed
- 2 teaspoons *garam masala*
- 2 pounds boneless chicken breasts, cut into strips
- 1 can light coconut milk
- 1 can tomato paste
- 1/2 teaspoon cayenne pepper
- 1 teaspoon dried coriander

- 1 tablespoon paprika
- 1 teaspoon turmeric powder
- 1 teaspoon cumin powder
- 1 1/2 teaspoons salt

Instructions

1. Heat olive oil in a skillet over medium flame and sauté the garlic for 1 minute. Add the garam masala and cook for another minute or until fragrant. Set aside.
2. Take the chicken in the Crock-Pot and add the garlic and garam masala mixture. Stir to coat the chicken meat.
3. Add the rest of the ingredients and cook on low for 7 hours.

Nutrition Information

Calories per serving: 520

Carbohydrates: 2.3 g

Protein: 32.7 g

Fat: 28 g

Sugar: 0 g

Sodium: 342 mg

Fiber: 0.8 g

14. Kashmiri Lamb Curry

Prep time: 40 minutes

Serves: 6

Ingredients

- 4 dried red chili peppers
- 3 long green fresh chili peppers
- 1 teaspoon cumin seeds
- 1 teaspoon garam masala
- 1 piece ginger root, peeled and grated
- 5 cloves garlic, crushed
- 1/4 cup unsweetened coconut meat, shredded
- 3 tomatoes, chopped
- 6 tablespoons vegetable oil
- 2 large onions, sliced
- 2 pounds lamb meat
- 1/2 teaspoon ground turmeric
- 1 cup plain yogurt
- 1/4 cup cilantro, chopped
- 1 cup water
- salt and pepper to taste

Instructions

1. Take the chilies, cumin seeds, garam masala, ginger, garlic, coconut, and tomatoes in a blender and pulse until smooth. Set aside.

2. In a skillet, heat vegetable oil and sauté the onions and lamb meat for 3 minutes.

3. Transfer the meat mixture in the Crock-Pot. Pour in chili paste mixture on top of the lamb.

4. Add the turmeric, yogurt, cilantro, and water. Season with salt and pepper.

5. Cook on low for 7 hours until tender.

Nutrition Information

Calories per serving: 489

Carbohydrates: 3 g

Protein: 25 g

Fat: 40 g

Sugar: 0 g

Sodium: 166 mg

Fiber: 2.5 g

15. Chicken with Bacon Gravy

Prep time: 35 minutes

Serves: 4

Ingredients

- 1 1/2 pounds chicken breasts, bones and skin removed
- 1/4 teaspoon pepper
- 1 teaspoon salt
- 1 teaspoon minced garlic
- 1 teaspoon dried thyme
- 6 slices of bacon, cooked and crumbled
- 1 1/2 cups water
- 2/3 cup heavy cream

Instructions

1. Take all ingredients except the heavy cream in the Crock-Pot.
2. Close the lid and cook on low for 6 hours.
3. Add the heavy cream and continue cooking for another hour.

Nutrition Information

Calories per serving: 359

Carbohydrates: 0.9 g

Protein: 21 g

Fat: 25 g

Sugar: 0 g

Sodium: 0 mg

Fiber: 0 g

16. Garlic Butter Chicken with Cream Cheese

Prep time: 20 minutes

Serves: 8

Ingredients

- 2 1/2 pounds chicken breast
- 1 stick butter, softened
- 8 cloves garlic, sliced in half
- 1 onion, sliced
- 1 1/2 teaspoon salt
- 8 ounces cream cheese
- 1 cup chicken stock

Instructions

1. Take the chicken in the Crock-Pot and add the butter.
2. Stir in the garlic and onions. Season with salt.
3. Cook on low for 6 hours.
4. Meanwhile, prepare the cream cheese sauce by mixing together cream cheese and chicken stock in a saucepan. Heat over medium flame and stir until the sauce has reduced.
5. Pour over the chicken.

Nutrition Information

Calories per serving: 463

Carbohydrates: 2 g

Protein: 22.4 g

Fat: 35 g

Sugar: 0 g

Sodium: 674 mg

Fiber: 0.6 g

17. Cheesy Adobo Chicken

Prep time: 30 minutes

Serves: 6

Ingredients

- 1 pound chicken breasts, bones removed but with skin on
- 1 tablespoon butter
- 1/2 cup tomatoes, sliced
- 2 tablespoons adobo sauce
- 1/2 cup milk
- 3/4 cup cheddar cheese, shredded

Instructions

1. Take all ingredients in the Crock-Pot.
2. Give a stir and cook on low for 8 hours.
3. Use a fork to shred the chicken.

Nutrition Information

Calories per serving: 493

Carbohydrates: 0 g

Protein: 25.8 g

Fat: 33.9 g

Sugar: 0 g

Sodium: 375 mg

Fiber: 0 g

18. Ketogenic Chicken Tikka Masala

Prep time: 25 minutes

Serves: 6

Ingredients

- 1 1/2 pounds chicken thighs, bone in and skin on
- 2 tablespoons olive oil
- 2 teaspoons onion powder
- 5 teaspoons garam masala
- 3 cloves of garlic
- 3 tablespoons tomato paste
- 1 inch gingerroot, grated
- 2 teaspoons smoked paprika
- 1 cup tomatoes, diced

- 1 cup coconut milk
- 1 cup heavy cream
- salt to taste
- fresh cilantro for garnish

Instructions

1. Take all ingredients except the cilantro in the Crock-Pot.
2. Mix everything until the spices are incorporated well.
3. Close the lid and cook on low for 8 hours.
4. Garnish with cilantro once cooked.

Nutrition Information

Calories per serving: 493

Carbohydrates: 4.3 g

Protein: 26.6 g

Fat: 41.2 g

Sugar: 1 g

Sodium: 457 mg

Fiber: 2 g

19. Balsamic Chicken Thighs

Prep time: 30 minutes

Serves: 8

Ingredients

- 1 teaspoon dried basil
- 2 teaspoons minced onion
- 1 teaspoon garlic powder
- 1/2 teaspoon salt
- 1/2 teaspoon black pepper
- 8 boneless chicken breasts
- 1 tablespoon extra-virgin olive oil
- 4 cloves garlic, minced
- 1/2 cup balsamic vinegar
- parsley for garnish

Instructions

1. In a small bowl, mix the dried basil, onion, garlic, salt, and pepper.
2. Rub the spice mixture onto the chicken. Set aside.
3. Take olive oil in the Crock-Pot and sprinkle minced garlic.
4. Arrange the chicken piece on top of the oil and garlic.
5. Pour balsamic vinegar.
6. Cook on low for 8 hours.
7. Garnish with parsley once cooked.

Nutrition Information

Calories per serving: 133

Carbohydrates: 5.6 g

Protein: 20.1 g

Fat: 4 g

Sugar: 3 g

Sodium: 832 mg

Fiber: 0.1 g

20. Chicken Lo Mein

Prep time: 40 minutes

Serves: 6

Ingredients

- 1 1/2 pounds chicken, sliced into strip
- 1 tablespoon coconut aminos
- 1/2 teaspoon sesame oil
- 1/2 teaspoon garlic paste
- 2 cloves garlic, minced
- 1 teaspoon ginger, minced
- 1 bunch bok choy, washed and sliced
- 12 ounces kelp noodles

- salt and pepper to taste
- 3/4 cup chicken broth
- 1 tablespoon rice vinegar
- 1 teaspoon red pepper chili flakes

Instructions

1. In a small bowl, mix the chicken, coconut aminos, sesame oil, and garlic paste. Let it marinate for 30 minutes inside the fridge.
2. Cook the marinated chicken in the Crock-Pot on high for 2 hours. Set aside.
3. Take the garlic, ginger, and bok choy at the bottom of the Crock-Pot. Add the chicken and kelp noodles on top. Season with salt and pepper to taste.
4. In a bowl, mix the chicken broth, rice vinegar, and red pepper flakes.
5. Pour over the chicken mixture and cook for 30 minutes on high.

Nutrition Information

Calories per serving: 174

Carbohydrates: 3.1 g

Protein: 24.5 g

Fat: 8.1 g

Sugar: 0.5 g

Sodium: 436 mg

Fiber: 1.6 g

21. Ethiopian Doro Watt Chicken

Prep time: 35 minutes

Serves: 6

Ingredients

- 1 teaspoon chili powder
- 1 teaspoon sweet paprika
- 1 tablespoon salt
- 1 teaspoon ground coriander
- 1/2 teaspoon ground ginger
- 1/8 teaspoon ground cardamom
- 1/8 teaspoon fenugreek powder
- 1/8 teaspoon nutmeg
- 1/8 teaspoon allspice
- 1 whole chicken, sliced into different parts
- 1/2 cup butter
- 2 large onions, chopped
- 1 clove of garlic, minced
- 8 hard-boiled eggs, shells removed

- 1/2 cup water

Instructions

1. Mix the first 9 ingredients in a bowl. Use this spice mix and rub it on the chicken parts. Let the chicken marinate for 30 minutes in the fridge.

2. Take the butter in the Crock-Pot and add the onion and garlic. Take the chicken pieces. Arrange the hard-boiled eggs randomly on top of the chicken.

3. Pour water.

4. Close the lid and cook on low for 8 hours.

Nutrition Information

Calories per serving: 315

Carbohydrates: 4 g

Protein: 19 g

Fat: 25 g

Sugar: 0 g

Sodium: 698 mg

Fiber: 0.8 g

Snack and Side Recipes

1. Crock-Pot Keto Chocolate Cake

Prep time: 20 minutes

Serves: 12

Ingredients

- 3/4 cup stevia sweetener
- 1 1/2 cups almond flour
- 1/4 cup protein powder, chocolate or vanilla flavor
- 2/3 cup cocoa powder, unsweetened
- 1/4 teaspoon baking powder
- 1/4 teaspoon salt
- 1/2 cup unsalted butter, melted
- 4 large eggs
- 3/4 cup heavy cream
- 1 teaspoon vanilla extract

Instructions

1. Grease the ceramic insert of the Crock-Pot.
2. In a bowl, mix the sweetener, almond flour, protein powder, cocoa powder, baking powder, and salt.
3. Add the butter, eggs, cream, and vanilla extract.
4. Pour the batter in the Crock-Pot and cook on low for 3 hours.
5. Allow it to cool before slicing.

Nutrition Information

Calories per serving: 253

Carbohydrates: 5.1 g

Protein: 17.3 g

Fat: 29.5 g

Sugar: 1.2 g

Sodium: 361 mg

Fiber: 2.4 g

2. *Keto Crock-Pot Chocolate Lava Cake*

Prep time: 30 minutes

Serves: 12

Ingredients

- 1 1/2 cups stevia sweetener, divided
- 1/2 cup almond flour
- 5 tablespoons unsweetened cocoa powder
- 1/2 teaspoon salt
- 1 teaspoon baking powder
- 3 whole eggs
- 3 egg yolks
- 1/2 cup butter, melted
- 1 teaspoon vanilla extract
- 2 cups hot water
- 4 ounces sugar-free chocolate chips

Instructions

1. Grease the inside of the Crock-Pot.

2. In a bowl, mix the stevia sweetener, almond flour, cocoa powder, salt, and baking powder.

3. In another bowl, mix the eggs, egg yolks, butter, and vanilla extract. Pour in the hot water.

4. Pour the wet ingredients to the dry ingredients and fold to create a batter.

5. Add the chocolate chips last.

6. Pour into the greased Crock-Pot and cook on low for 3 hours.

7. Allow to cool before serving.

Nutrition Information

Calories per serving: 157

Carbohydrates: 5.5 g

Protein: 10.6 g

Fat: 13 g

Sugar: 0.2 g

Sodium: 155 mg

Fiber: 2.6 g

3. Lemon Crock-Pot Cake

Prep time: 15 minutes

Serves: 8

Ingredients

- 1/2 cup coconut flour
- 1 1/2 cups almond flour
- 3 tablespoons stevia sweetener
- 2 teaspoons baking powder
- 1/2 teaspoon xanthan gum
- 1/2 cup whipping cream
- 1/2 cup butter, melted
- 1 tablespoon juice, freshly squeezed
- zest from one large lemon
- 2 eggs

Instructions

1. Grease the inside of the Crock-Pot with butter or cooking spray.
2. Mix together coconut flour, almond flour, stevia, baking powder, and xanthan gum in a bowl.
3. In another bowl, combine the whipping cream, butter, lemon juice, lemon zest, and eggs. Mix until well combined.
4. Pour the wet ingredients to the dry ingredients gradually and fold to create a smooth batter.
5. Spread the batter in the Crock-Pot and cook on low for 3 hours or until a toothpick inserted in the middle comes out clean.

Nutrition Information

Calories per serving: 350

Carbohydrates: 11.1 g

Protein: 17.6 g

Fat: 32.6 g

Sugar: 0.9 g

Sodium: 224 mg

Fiber: 4.9 g

4. Keto Basic Vanilla Cake in a Crock-Pot

Prep time: 25 minutes

Serves: 12

Ingredients

- 1 1/2 cups almond flour
- 3/4 cup stevia sweetener
- 2/3 cup protein powder, vanilla powder
- 1/4 teaspoon salt
- 2 teaspoons baking powder
- 1/2 cup unsalted butter, melted
- 3/4 cup heavy cream
- 4 large eggs
- 1 teaspoon vanilla extract

Instructions

1. Grease the insert of the Crock-Pot with cooking spray.

2. In a bowl, mix the almond flour, sweetener, protein powder, salt, and baking powder.

3. In another bowl, combine the butter, heavy cream, eggs, and vanilla extract.

4. Pour the wet ingredients to the dry ingredients and fold to create a smooth batter.

5. Pour into the greased Crock-Pot.

6. Cook on low for 3 hours.

7. Let it cool before serving.

Nutrition Information

Calories per serving: 162

Carbohydrates: 4.1 g

Protein: 11.6 g

Fat: 12.3 g

Sugar: 2.3 g

Sodium: 154 mg

Fiber: 0.5 g

5. Mocha Pudding Cake

Prep time: 60 minutes

Serves: 6

Ingredients

- 3/4 cup butter, cut into chunks
- 2 ounces unsweetened chocolate, chopped
- 1/2 cup heavy cream
- 2 tablespoons instant coffee
- 1 teaspoon vanilla extract
- 1/3 cup almond flour
- 4 tablespoons cocoa powder, unsweetened
- 1/8 teaspoon salt
- 5 large eggs
- 2/3 cup stevia sweetener

Instructions

1. Grease the Crock-Pot pot with cooking spray or butter.
2. In a double boiler, melt the butter and unsweetened chocolate over medium heat. Once melted, remove from heat and allow to cool.
3. In a small bowl, combine the heavy cream, coffee, and vanilla extract.
4. In another bowl, combine the almond flour, cocoa powder, and salt.
5. Beat the eggs in a large bowl and add the stevia sweetener until slightly thickened or until it turns pale yellow.

6. To the egg mixture, pour in the melted chocolate. Whisk until combined. Add the flour mixture gradually while continuously whisking.

7. Pour in the coffee mixture last. Whisk until combined.

8. Pour the batter into the Crock-Pot.

9. Place a paper towel on top of the Crock-Pot before closing the lid.

10. Cook on low for 3 hours.

Nutrition Information

Calories per serving: 414

Carbohydrates: 3.8 g

Protein: 10.9 g

Fat: 38.9 g

Sugar: 13 g

Sodium: 542 mg

Fiber: 0.9 g

6. Cinnamon Blondie Pecan Bars

Prep time: 55 minutes

Serves: 16

Ingredients

- 1 cup stevia sweetener

- 6 tablespoons unsalted butter, melted
- 3 large eggs
- 2 teaspoons vanilla extract
- 1 1/2 cups almond flour
- 1/4 teaspoon salt
- 1 tablespoon cinnamon
- 1 teaspoon baking powder
- 2 tablespoons unsalted butter
- 1/4 cup heavy whipping cream
- 1 cup pecans, chopped

Instructions

1. Grease the Crock-Pot with butter.
2. In a bowl, combine the stevia sweetener and melted butter. Add in the eggs and vanilla extract.
3. Use a hand mixer to combine the ingredients.
4. In another bowl, combine the almond flour, salt, baking powder, and cinnamon.
5. Mix the wet ingredients to the dry ingredients until combined.
6. Pour the dough in the Crock-Pot and press to form a dense bar.
7. Cook on low for 3 hours.

8. Meanwhile, mix the butter, whipping cream and pecans in a saucepan. Allow to boil and reduce slightly.

9. Once the bars are cooked, pour over the pecan sauce.

Nutrition Information

Calories per serving: 190.6

Carbohydrates: 1.9 g

Protein: 4.42 g

Fat: 20.56 g

Sugar: 0.5 g

Sodium: 163 mg

Fiber: 0 g

7. Crock-Pot Dark Chocolate Cake

Prep time: 40 minutes

Serves: 10

Ingredients

- 1 cup almond flour
- 1/2 cup cocoa powder
- 1/2 cup stevia sweetener
- 3 tablespoons whey protein powder, unflavored
- 1 1/2 teaspoons baking powder

- 1/4 teaspoon salt

- 3 large eggs

- 2/3 cup unsweetened almond milk

- 6 tablespoons butter, melted

- 3/4 teaspoon vanilla extract

- 1/3 cup sugar-free chocolate chips

Instructions

1. Grease the Crock-Pot with butter.

2. In a medium bowl, whisk the almond flour, cocoa powder, stevia powder, and whey protein. Add in the baking powder and salt.

3. In another bowl, combine the eggs, almond milk, butter, and vanilla extract.

4. Pour the wet ingredients to the dry ingredients and whisk until the batter is smooth.

5. Add the chocolate chips last.

6. Pour the batter in the Crock-Pot and bake on low for 3 hours.

Nutrition Information

Calories per serving: 205

Carbohydrates: 8.42 g

Protein: 7.37 g

Fat: 16.79 g

Sugar: 0.3 g

Sodium: 230 mg

Fiber: 4.1 g

8. Easy Crock-Pot Cheesecake

Prep time: 35 minutes

Serves: 6

Ingredients

- 3 (8-ounce) cream cheese, room temperature
- 1 cup stevia sweetener
- 3 eggs
- 1/2 tablespoon vanilla extract

Instructions

1. Grease the Crock-Pot with butter.
2. In a mixing bowl, mix the cream cheese and stevia sweetener.
3. Use a hand mixer to mix everything.
4. Add the eggs and vanilla extract.
5. Pour the mixture into the Crock-Pot and cook on low for 3 hours.

Nutrition Information

Calories per serving: 264

Carbohydrates: 3 g

Protein: 9.1 g

Fat: 15.8 g

Sugar: 2.6 g

Sodium: 157 mg

Fiber: 0 g

Dessert Recipes

1. Pumpkin Pecan Pie Ice Cream (4 one-cup servings)

Or for extra decadence, one can add 3–4 ounces cream cheese to this recipe.

Ingredients

- 1/2 cup cottage cheese
- 1/2 cup pumpkin puree
- 1 teaspoon pumpkin spice
- 2 cups coconut milk
- 1/2 teaspoon xantham gum
- 3 large egg yolks
- 1/3 cup erythritol
- 20 drops liquid stevia

Nutrient intake per serving:

Carbs: 4.3 g

Fat: 22.3 g

Protein: 6.5 g

Calories: 248

- 1 teaspoon maple extract

- ½ cup pecans, toasted and chopped

- 2 tablespoons salted butter

Instructions

- Chop the toasted pecans and put on the stove with butter. Leave it over low heat until the butter turns brown. In case you don't have toasted pecans, place in a pan and toast over low heat for between 7 and 10 minutes.

- Place all the ingredients into a container that can accommodate the immersion blender.

- Use your immersion blender to blend all the ingredients together into a mixture that is smooth.

- Add the mixture to your ice-cream machine.

- Once your butter turns brown and the pecans have soaked up some of the butter, place inside the ice-cream machine.

- Follow the churning instructions as per your ice-cream manufacturer's instructions.

2. Ketogenic Amaretti Cookies (16 cookies)

These are delicate and sweet. Each one is soft and full of almond and fruity flavors. This recipe uses strawberry jam.

Ingredients

- 1 cup almond flour
- 2 tablespoons coconut flour
- ½ teaspoon baking powder
- 1/4 teaspoon baking powder
- 1/4 teaspoon cinnamon
- Half a teaspoon of salt
- 1/2 cup erythritol
- 2 large eggs
- 4 tablespoons coconut oil
- 1/2 teaspoon vanilla extract
- 1/2 teaspoon almond extract
- 2 tablespoons sugar-free jam
- 1 tablespoon organic shredded coconut

Nutrient intake per serving:

Carbs: 1.2 g

Fat: 7.9 g

Protein: 2.4 g

Calories: 86

Instructions

- Preheat the oven to 350°F. Mix all the dry ingredients and whisk.
- Add in the wet ingredients and mix well. Use a whisk or hand mixer.

- Form the cookies on a parchment-paper-lined baking sheet. Add an indent at the middle of each cookie using your finger or the back of a measuring spoon.

- Bake for about 15 minutes or until the cookies turn golden or crack slightly.

- Let the cookies cool on a wire rack and fill each indent with sugar-free jam.

- Lastly, sprinkle some shredded coconut on top of each cookie.

- Dish out and serve.

These bars are easy to make and can be frozen or refrigerated depending on what you need.

3. No-Bake Coconut Cashew Bars (8 servings)

Ingredients

- 1 cup almond flour
- 1/4 cup melted butter
- 1/4 cup sugar-free maple syrup
- 1 teaspoon cinnamon
- a pinch of salt
- 1/2 cup cashews
- 1/4 cup shredded coconut

Nutrient intake per serving:

Carbs: 4 g

Fat: 17.6 g

Protein: 4 g

Calories: 189

Instructions

- Mix the melted butter and almond flour in a large bowl.

- Add cinnamon, salt, and sugar-free maple syrup and mix properly.

- You then add the shredded coconut and mix again.

- Roughly chop 1/2 cup of cashews, whether raw or roasted. Add to the coconut cashew bar dough. Mix well.

- Line a baking dish with parchment paper and spread the coconut cashew bar dough in an even layer. You can add some more shredded coconut and cinnamon on top.

- Place them in the refrigerator and chill for at least two hours. However, overnight is recommended. As soon as they are chilled, slice them into bars. Serve and enjoy!

4. Ketogenic Chocolate-Covered Macaroons (12 macaroons)

These macaroons are sweet with a nice coconut, almond, and chocolate flavor.

Ingredients

- 1 cup unsweetened shredded coconut
- 1 large white egg
- 1/4 cup erythritol
- 1/2 teaspoon almond extract
- a pinch of salt
- 20 grams sugar-free chocolate
- 2 tablespoons coconut oil

Nutrient intake per serving:

Carbs: 1 g

Fat: 7.3 g

Protein: 1 g

Calories: 73

Instructions

- Preheat the oven to 350°F and spread a cup of shredded and unsweetened coconut into a thin layer on a parchment-paper-lined baking sheet. As soon as the oven is hot enough, place the coconut in to toast up a little for about five minutes.

- As the coconut toasts, beat the egg white until it's foamy.

- Add the erythritol and a pinch of salt as you continue to mix.

- You then add the almond extract for a twist on normal coconut macaroons.

- Once the coconut flakes have toasted and cooled, add them in and fold everything together.

- Use an ice-cream scoop or your hands to tightly pack little balls of macaroon batter and gently place them on a parchment-paper-lined baking sheet. Bake until they are golden. This should take around 15 minutes.

- As they bake, make the chocolate drizzle by melting coconut oil and the sugar-free chocolate. Continuously stir to make sure the chocolate doesn't burn.

- When the macaroons are out of the oven, drizzle your chocolate over each one of them.

5. Ketogenic Chocolate Peanut Butter Tarts (4 servings)

Ingredients

Crust:

- 1/4 cup flaxseeds
- 2 tablespoons almond flour
- 1 tablespoon erythritol
- 1 large egg white

Top layer:

- 1 medium avocado
- 4 tablespoons cocoa powder
- 1/4 cup erythritol
- 1/2 teaspoon vanilla extract
- 1/2 teaspoon cinnamon
- 2 tablespoons heavy cream

Middle layer:

- 4 tablespoons peanut butter
- 2 tablespoons butter

Instructions

- Preheat the oven to 350°F. Make your crust by grinding up 1/4 cup flaxseeds until they are finely ground.

Nutrient intake per serving:

Carbs: 3.9 g

Fat: 26.8 g

Protein: 9.8 g

Calories: 305

- Add the rest of the crust ingredients to the ground flaxseeds. Blend until well mixed.

- Press the crust mixture into the tart pans and up the sides. Bake for about 8 minutes until set.

- As the crust bakes, prepare the top layer by mixing all the ingredients in a blender and blend until smooth and creamy.

- After removing the crusts from the oven, let them cool as you prepare your peanut butter layer. Melt the peanut butter and butter in the microwave or a small pan over the stove until well mixed and soft.

- Pour the melted layer of peanut butter onto the tart crusts and place in the fridge for half an hour until set.

- As soon as the top of the peanut butter layer is set, add the chocolate avocado layer on top. Smooth it out and refrigerate for an hour.

6. Peaches and Cream Dessert

Peaches and cream dessert is a delicious summer delicacy and fit perfectly in the keto diet with the right calories count.

Prep time: 10 minutes

Ingredients

- 4 tablespoons unsalted butter, softened
- 6 ounces softened cream cheese
- 1 cup frozen peaches, warmed lightly
- 3/4 scoop peaches and cream ketone supplement
- 3 1/2 tablespoon fruit sweetener, separated

Nutrient intake per cookie:

- Fat: 43 g
- Carbs: 4.21 g
- Net carbs: 0.9 g
- Protein: 0.5 g

Instructions

- In a medium-sized bowl with a hand mixer, mix butter, cream cheese, peaches, peaches and cream ketone supplement, and 3 tablespoons of monk fruit sweetener until well-combined.
- Scoop mixture into a silicone mold. Top each fat bomb with remaining monk fruit sweetener.
- Place mold in the freezer and freeze for 4 hours.
- Once frozen, remove fat bombs from silicone mold and enjoy!
- Freeze time: 4 hours.

Nutrition

Calories: 43

Fat: 4.2

Carbohydrates: 1

Net carbs: 0.9

Protein: 0.5

7. Lemon Cashew Cookies

Lemon cashew cookies are low in carbohydrates and are a nutritious dessert for the keto diet, but because cashews are high in carbs, use only raw cashew butter with no added sugar. In place of cashew nuts, you can also use macadamia nuts, which are high in fat (80% monounsaturated) and are rich in antioxidants, minerals, and vitamins.

Prep time: 10 minutes

Cook time: 12 minutes

Total time: 22 minutes

Yield: 12

Category: snacks

Cuisine: American

Ingredients

- 1 cup cashew butter
- 2 eggs
- zest of 1 lemon
- juice of 1 lemon
- 1/2 teaspoon vanilla extract
- 6–10 drops liquid stevia (or 1/4 teaspoon powdered stevia)
- 1/4 teaspoon baking soda

Nutrient intake per cookie:
Calories: 140 g
Sugar: 3 g
Fat: 9 g
Carbohydrates: 4 g
Protein: 4 g

Instructions

- Preheat oven to 350°F.
- Wash the lemon and dry it thoroughly. Use a fine grater to zest the lemon rind into a large bowl. Be sure to get the entire colorful outer layer of the lemon. Then cut open the lemon and squeeze the juice into the bowl being careful not to let any seeds in the bowl.
- Add the cashew butter, eggs, vanilla, baking soda, and stevia to the bowl and mix with a fork or spoon until all of the ingredients are fully blended.
- The consistency will be like a thick, viscous batter, which is a bit thicker than nut butter but a bit thinner than the usual cookie dough. Take 12 small heaps of the batter and place onto a cookie sheet, shaping into a cookie shape.
- Bake at 350°F for about 10–15 minutes. Let cool before serving.

Tips about the Desserts and Ingredients

Benefits of peaches:

- Peaches have 17% daily recommended value in vitamin C per serving, which boosts immunity.
- Peaches are low in saturated fat and cholesterol.
- They are a good source of vitamin E, vitamin K, niacin, and copper.
- They have vitamin A, which offers B-carotenes that convert to retinol, which is essential for sharp eyesight

- They are abundant in potassium to aid in the digestion of food, heart-rate regulation, and the lowering of blood pressure.
- Iron in peaches is required for red blood cell formation.
- Magnesium helps to prevent stress and anxiety and keeps the nervous system calm.
- The combination of phosphorous and calcium strengthens bones and teeth.
- Phenolic compounds containing anti-inflammatory and anti-obesity properties help fight metabolic syndromes.

Dinner Recipes

1. Low-Carb Walnut-Crusted Salmon (2 servings)

In the ketogenic diet, fatty fish has been proven to lower levels of cholesterol and aid with the overall health. This recipe is easy to prepare and super tasty. It takes under 15 minutes to prepare.

Nutrient intake per serving:
Carbs: 3 g
Fat: 43 g
Protein: 20 g
Calories: 373

Ingredients

- 1/2 cup of walnuts
- 2 tablespoons sugar-free maple syrup
- 1/2 tablespoon Dijon mustard
- 1/4 teaspoon dill
- 2 (3-ounce) salmon fillets
- 1 tablespoon olive oil
- salt and pepper

Instructions

- Preheat the oven to 350°F. Add half a cup of walnuts to the food processor.
- Add two tablespoons of maple syrup and the spices.
- Add a tablespoon of mustard.
- Pulse this in the food processor until it is paste-like.

- Heat a pan or skillet with a tablespoon of oil until very hot. Thoroughly dry the salmon fillets and place them skin-down in the pan. Let it sear for about 3 minutes, undisturbed.
- As it sears, add the walnut mixture to the top side of the salmon fillets.
- After that, transfer them to an oven and bake for about 8 minutes.
- Serve with fresh spinach and enjoy. You can sprinkle a little bit of smoked paprika.

2. Keto Hot-Chili Soup (4 servings)

Ingredients

- 1 teaspoon coriander seeds
- 2 tablespoons olive oil
- 2 sliced chili peppers
- 2 cups chicken broth
- 2 cups water
- 1 teaspoon turmeric
- 1/2 teaspoon ground cumin
- 4 tablespoons tomato paste
- 16 ounces chicken thighs
- 2 tablespoons butter
- 1 medium avocado
- 2 ounces queso fresco
- 4 tablespoons fresh chopped cilantro
- juice from half a lime
- salt and pepper

Nutrient intake per serving:
Carbs: 5.8 g
Fat: 27.8 g
Protein: 28 g
Calories: 396

Instructions

- Cut and set the chicken thighs to cook in an oiled pan. Season it with salt and pepper. You then leave it aside to rest.
- In 2 tablespoons of olive oil, heat up the coriander seeds to release more flavor.

- Once they are fragrant, add in the sliced chili peppers to add their flavor to the oil.
- You then add in the broth and water. Let it simmer and season. Add turmeric, ground cumin, and salt and pepper to taste.
- As the soup simmers, add in the tomato paste and butter. Stir so that it melts and mixes. Let the soup simmer for between 5 and 10 minutes.
- Lower the heat on the stove and the juice from half the lime.
- Place 4 ounces of chicken thighs into the bottom of the bowl so that you are able to pour soup over it.
- Ladle the soup for serving. Garnish with a quarter of an avocado into each bowl, 1/2 ounce of queso fresco, and cilantro.

3. Slow-Cooker Ketogenic Chicken Tikka Masala (5 servings)
Ingredients

- 1 (1/2-pound) chicken thighs, bone in, skin on
- 1 pound chicken thighs, boneless, skinless
- 2 tablespoons olive oil
- 2 teaspoons onion powder
- 3 cloves minced garlic
- 1 inch grated gingerroot
- 3 tablespoons tomato paste
- 5 teaspoons garam masala
- 2 teaspoons smoked paprika
- 4 teaspoons of kosher salt
- 10 ounces diced tomatoes, canned
- 1 cup heavy cream
- 1 cup coconut milk
- fresh chopped cilantro
- 1 teaspoon guar gum

Instructions

Nutrient intake per serving:
Carbs: 5.8 g
Fat: 41.2 g
Protein: 26 g
Calories: 493

- Debone the chicken on the bone-in chicken thighs. Chop all the chicken pieces into bite-sized pieces. Ensure that you keep the skin for the pieces that have it.
- Add the chicken to a slow cooker and grate an inch of ginger over the top.
- Add all the dry spices into the slow cooker and mix properly.
- Add canned diced tomatoes and tomato paste into the slow cooker and mix well once more.
- Finally, add 1/2 cup of coconut milk and mix well. Cook over low heat for 6 hours or 3 hours over high heat.
- Once the slow cooker is over, add the remainder of the coconut milk, heavy cream, and guar gum and mix well into the chicken. This will help the curry thicken nicely.
- Serve over cauliflower rice or a veggie of your choice.

4. Barbecue Bacon Cheeseburger Waffles (2 servings)

This meal is dense with calories.

Ingredients

Waffles:

- 5 ounces cheddar cheese
- 2 large eggs
- 1 cup cauliflower crumbles
- 1/4 teaspoon garlic powder
- 1/4 teaspoon onion powder
- 4 tablespoons almond flour
- 3 tablespoons Parmesan cheese
- salt and pepper

The topping:

- 4 ounces ground beef
- 4 slices of chopped bacon
- 4 tablespoons sugar-free barbecue sauce
- 1 1/2 ounces cheddar cheese

Nutrient intake per serving:
Carbs: 3 g
Fat: 29.8 g
Protein: 18.8 g
Calories: 354

- salt and pepper

Instructions

- Shred 3 ounces of cheese. You will use half for the waffle and half on top.
- Measure out the cauliflower crumbles over a scale or use a cup.
- Mix in half of the cheddar cheese, Parmesan cheese, eggs, almond flour, and spices.
- Slice the bacon thinly over medium to high heat.
- As soon as the bacon is partially cooked, add in the beef.
- Add any excess grease from the pan into the waffle mixture that you set aside.
- Use an immersion blender to blend the waffle mixture into a paste that is thick.
- Add half of the mixture to the waffle iron and cook until crisp. Repeat for the second waffle.
- As the waffles cook, add in the sugar-free barbecue sauce to the bacon and ground mixture of the beef.
- Assemble the waffles together by adding half of the ground beef mixture and half of the remaining cheddar cheese to the top of the waffle
- Broil for about two minutes until the cheese is nicely melted over the top.

- Serve immediately. You may slice up green onion to sprinkle over the top.

5. *Bacon Cheeseburger Casserole (6 servings)*

Ingredients

- 1 pound ground beef
- 3 slices of bacon
- 1/2 cup of almond flour
- 256 grams cauliflower, riced
- 1 tablespoon psyllium husk powder
- 1/2 teaspoon garlic powder
- 1/2 teaspoon onion powder
- 2 tablespoons reduced sugar ketchup
- 1 tablespoon Dijon mustard
- 2 tablespoons mayonnaise
- 3 large eggs
- 4 ounces cheddar cheese
- salt and pepper

Nutrient intake per serving:
Carbs: 3.6 g
Fat: 35.5 g
Protein: 32.2 g
Calories: 478

Instructions

- Preheat the oven to 350°F. Put rice cauliflower in the food processor and add dry ingredients. Mix well.
- Put bacon and ground beef in the food processor until crumbly. Cook over medium to high heat. Season with salt and pepper.
- Shred the cheese as the meat cooks. Once the meat is done, mix all the ingredients in a large bowl and add half of the cheddar cheese.
- Add eggs, mayo, ketchup, and mustard to the mixture. Use a fork or hands to mix everything well.
- Press the mixture into a 9×9 baking pan lined with parchment paper. You then top with the other half of the cheddar cheese.
- Place on the top rack and bake for 25–30 minutes. For additional crisp on top, broil for around 3 minutes or until browned.

- Remove from oven and let it cool for between five and ten minutes.
- Slice and serve with additional toppings.

6. Shrimp Stir-Fry

Shrimp stir-fry is a great low-carb, high-fat keto meal that you can have ready within half an hour—shrimp healthily sautéed in bacon. Serve with a keto-friendly vegetable like cauliflower rice as a side dish to beef up nutrients. The portion of fat used is keto healthy and the bacon boosts the fat content, which ensures sufficient fat stores for fuel.

Ingredients

- 16 ounces (or 1 pound) shrimps, peeled with tail on
- 2 inches gingerroot
- 4 stalks scallion or green onion
- 2 garlic cloves
- 4 baby bella mushrooms
- 1 inch lemon rind
- 2 teaspoon sea salt (or to taste)
- 3 tablespoons bacon fat
- 12 ounces frozen cauliflower rice
- 2 tablespoons MCT oil
- coconut aminos
- sesame seeds
- chili flakes

Nutrient intake per serving:
Calories: 357
Fat: 24.8
Carbs: 9
Protein: 24.7

Instructions

- Preheat oven to 400°F.
- Drizzle MCT oil liberally on cauliflower on a sheet pan and sprinkle the salt.
- Place in the oven once it reaches 400°F and cook for 10 minutes.
- Cut scallion into pieces of about 1 inch. Peel enough lemon rind. Slice garlic and ginger.

- Sauté the onions, ginger, and garlic in bacon fat on medium heat in a large skillet until they are aromatic and soft.
- Once they are soft, add the shrimp and sauté. Keep stirring until the shrimps turn pink and are coiled.
- Add coconut aminos and more salt (if you want). Keep stirring for 3 minutes and then turn off the heat.
- Serve the sautéed shrimp over the cauliflower rice and garnish with chili flakes, green onion, and sesame seeds.

7. Bone Broth

Broth soup is nutrient-rich. It boosts immunity and reduces inflammation. Simmer animal bone in water infused with herbs and vinegar to melt out the collagen in the bone and marrow.

Prep time: 1 hour

Cook: 23 hours

Ingredients

- 4 pounds animal bone pastured (or 3 pounds pastured whole chicken)
- 10 cups filtered water (or as you deem enough)
- 2 tablespoons peppercorns
- 1 lemon
- 3 tablespoons turmeric
- 1 teaspoon salt
- 2 tablespoons apple cider vinegar
- 3 bay leaves (or as you want)

Nutrient intake per cup serving:
Calories: 70
Sugar: 0
Fat: 4
Carbs: 1
Protein: 6

Instructions

- Preheat oven to 400°F.
- Roast bones or chicken for 45 minutes on a sheet pan and sprinkle salt.
- Transfer to a slow cooker or an electric pressure cooker.
- Add apple cider vinegar, bay leaves, peppercorns, and water.

- Simmer on low for 24–48 hours. If pressure cooking, do high for 2 hours then turn to slow cook for 12 hours.
- After that, sieve the broth over a large bowl.
- Discard everything else other than the strained broth.
- Divide the broth into three bowls or jars each with 2 cups.
- Add a teaspoon of turmeric and a slice or 2 of lemon to each of the 3 containers.
- Refrigerate and eat within 5 days.
- Warm on low heat.

8. *Baked Cauliflower with Bacon and Cheese*

This is a satiating meal high in fat and low on carbs combining cauliflower nutrient with cheese and bacon.

Prep time: 15 minutes

Cook time: 45 minutes

Total time: 1 hour

Yield: 4

Ingredients

- 1 large head cauliflower, cut into florets
- 2 tablespoon butter
- 1 cup heavy cream
- 2 ounces cream cheese
- 1 1/4 cups shredded sharp cheddar cheese, separated
- salt and pepper to taste
- six slices bacon, cooked and crumbled
- 1/4 cup chopped green onions

Nutrient intake per serving:
Calories: 498
Fat: 45
Carbs: 5.8
Net carbs: 4.1
Protein: 13.9

Instructions

- Preheat oven to 350°F.
- In a large pot of boiling water, blanch cauliflower florets for 2 minutes. Drain cauliflower.

- In a medium pot, melt together butter, heavy cream, cream cheese, 1 cup of shredded cheddar cheese, salt, and pepper until well-combined.
- In a baking dish, add cauliflower florets, cheese sauce, all but 1 tablespoon crumbled bacon, and all but 1 tablespoon green onions. Stir together.
- Top with remaining shredded cheddar cheese, crumbled bacon, and green onions.
- Bake until cheese is bubbly and golden and cauliflower is soft, about 30 minutes.
- Serve immediately and enjoy!

9. Miracle Noodle Stuffed with Chicken

Miracle noodle stuffed with chicken is an effortless easy dinner fix—a dish combining different foods in one. Miracle noodles, also known as Shirataki noodles, are zero-carb Japanese noodles. Depending on the type of miracle noodle, they are very low carb to no carb. They are made of 3% glucomannan fiber, which slows down glucose absorption (thus blood sugar regulating), and 97% water.

Cook time: 25–35 minutes

Total time: 45 minutes

Ingredients

- 1 pack miracle noodle angel hair pasta
- 1 tablespoon avocado oil
- 2 cups spinach
- 2 ounces mozzarella cheese
- 1 pound boneless skinless chicken breast
- 1 teaspoon salt
- 1 teaspoon pepper

Nutrient intake per serving:

1 chicken breast (6 ounces)

Calories: 363

Fat: 13 g

Carbohydrates:

Net carbs: 2.3 g

Fiber: 1.7 g

Protein: 60 g

- 1 teaspoon white pepper

Instructions

- Preheat oven to 400°F.
- While oven is heating up, prepare the miracle noodles by draining them and adding them to a pot of boiling water. Let it simmer in water for 10 minutes.
- While the miracle noodles are simmering, sautée spinach and avocado oil in a pan on medium heat.
- Place chicken on cutting board and cut slices in them hasselback-style, enough room to stuff with pasta and spinach.
- Drain the miracle noodles and add to the spinach pan. Mix in cheese. Mix all together.
- Add spoonfuls of miracle noodles, spinach, and cheese to the pockets cut in the chicken breasts.
- Once all the pockets are stuffed, place the chicken on a baking sheet covered with parchment paper.
- Place in the oven to bake for 25–35 minutes or until fully cooked.

10. Easy White Turkey Chili

Preparation: 5 minutes

Cook time: 15 minutes

Total time: 20 minutes

Ingredients

- 1 pound organic ground turkey (or ground beef, lamb, or pork)

- 2 cups riced cauliflower
- 2 tablespoon coconut oil
- 1/2 a Vidalia onion
- 2 garlic cloves
- 2 cups full-fat coconut milk (or heavy cream)
- 1 tablespoon mustard
- 1 teaspoon salt, black pepper, thyme, celery salt, garlic powder

Nutrient intake per cup serving:
Calories: 388
Fat: 30.5
Carbs: 5.5
Protein: 28.8

Instructions

- In a large pot, heat the coconut oil.
- In the meantime, mince the onion and garlic. Add it to the hot oil.
- Stir for 2–3 minutes then add in the ground turkey.
- Break up with the spatula and stir constantly until crumbled.
- Add in the seasoning mix and riced cauliflower and stir well.
- Once the meat is browned add in the coconut milk, bring to a simmer and reduce for 5–8 minutes, stirring often.
- At this point, it's ready to serve, or you can let it reduce by half until thick and serve as a dip.
- Mix in shredded cheese for an extra thick sauce.

Topping suggestions:

- Avocado
- Jalapenos
- Bacon
- Shredded aged cheddar cheese
- Cherry tomatoes
- Hot sauce

11. *Bacon Cheddar Broccoli Salad*

Prep time: 35 minutes

Serves: 6

Ingredients

- 6 slices raw bacon, chopped
- 1 bunch steamed broccoli, cut into small florets
- 3/4 cup mayonnaise
- 2 tablespoons apple cider vinegar
- 3 packets stevia powder
- 1/2 cup cheddar cheese
- 1/4 cup onion, chopped
- 1/4 cup sunflower seeds, roasted

Instructions

1. Take a parchment paper on the bottom of the Crock-Pot. Take the bacon in the Crock-Pot.
2. Cook on low for 8 hours or until the bacon is crispy.
3. Take the bacon in a bowl and add the steamed broccoli.
4. In another bowl, add the mayonnaise, apple cider vinegar, and stevia powder. Mix well.
5. Pour over the bacon and broccoli and toss to mix.
6. Add the cheddar cheese, onion, and sunflower seeds.

Nutrition Information

Calories per serving: 231

Carbohydrates: 8.1 g

Protein: 16 g

Fat: 15.3 g

Sugar: 2.4 g

Sodium: 751 mg

Fiber: 3 g

12. Chicken Yellow Curry

Prep time: 40 minutes

Serves: 6

Ingredients

- 1 1/2 pounds chicken breasts, skin and bones removed

- 6 cups mixed vegetables (preferably broccoli and cauliflower)
- 1 can full-fat coconut milk
- 1 cup crushed tomatoes
- 1 tablespoon cumin
- 2 teaspoons ground coriander
- 2 teaspoons ground ginger
- 2 teaspoons ground ginger powder
- 1 teaspoon cinnamon
- 1/2 teaspoon cayenne pepper
- 1 cup water
- salt to taste

Instructions

1. Take the chicken and vegetables in the Crock-Pot.
2. Add the rest of the ingredients and stir to mix everything.
3. Close the lid and cook on low for 6 hours.

Nutrition Information

Calories per serving: 425

Carbohydrates: 3 g

Protein: 23 g

Fat: 31.4 g

Sugar: 0 g

Sodium: 371.4 mg

Fiber: 0.9 g

13. Thai Whole Chicken Soup

Prep time: 25 minutes

Serves: 10

Ingredients

- 1 whole chicken
- 1 stalk lemongrass, cut into chunks
- 20 fresh basil leaves
- 5 thick slices of ginger

- 1 tablespoon salt (or more if needed)
- 1 lime, sliced

Instructions

1. Take the whole chicken inside the Crock-Pot.
2. Surround it with lemongrass stalks, 10 basil leaves, and ginger.
3. Fill the Crock-Pot with water until the maximum line. Season with salt.
4. Cook on low for 10 hours or until the chicken is tender.
5. Serve with lime and the remaining basil leaves.

Nutrition Information

Calories per serving: 475

Carbohydrates: 2 g

Protein: 42 g

Fat: 12 g

Sugar: 0 g

Sodium: 278 mg

Fiber: 0.5 g

14. Lemongrass and Coconut Chicken Drumsticks

Prep time: 15 minutes

Serves: 6

Ingredients

- 10 drumsticks, skin removed
- salt and pepper to taste
- 1 stalk lemongrass, cut into 5-inch-long sticks
- 3 tablespoon extra-virgin olive oil
- 1 thumb-sized ginger
- 4 cloves garlic, minced
- 2 tablespoons fish sauce
- 1 cup coconut milk
- 3 tablespoons coconut aminos
- 1 teaspoon five-spice powder

- 1 large onion, sliced thinly
- 1/4 cup fresh scallions, chopped

Instructions

1. Take the chicken drumstick in a bowl and season with salt and pepper. Set aside.
2. In a blender, take the lemongrass, oil ginger, garlic, fish sauce, coconut milk, aminos, and five-spice powder. Blend until a smooth paste is formed.
3. Pour the paste or sauce into the marinated chicken and mix well. Allow it to marinate for another 2 hours.
4. Take the onion in the Crock-Pot and add the marinated chicken.
5. Cook on low for 8 hours.
6. Sprinkle with scallions on top.

Nutrition Information

Calories per serving: 528

Carbohydrates: 2 g

Protein: 32 g

Fat: 27 g

Sugar: 0 g

Sodium: 325 mg

Fiber: 0.8 g

15. Crock-Pot Beef Stroganoff

Prep time: 30 minutes

Serves: 8

Ingredients

- 2 pounds beef stew meat
- 2 teaspoons salt
- 1/2 teaspoon black pepper
- 1 teaspoon garlic powder
- 3 tablespoons extra-virgin olive oil

- 2 teaspoons paprika
- 1 teaspoon thyme
- 1 teaspoon onion powder
- 8 ounces mushrooms, sliced
- 1 small onion, sliced
- 1/3 cup coconut cream
- 2 teaspoons vinegar

Instructions

1. Season the beef stew meat with salt and pepper. Add the garlic powder, oil, paprika, thyme, and onion powder. Stir to mix all ingredients. Let the beef marinate for 2 hours inside the fridge.
2. Take the mushrooms and onion in the Crock-Pot and take the seasoned beef on top.
3. Close the lid and cook on low for 8 hours.
4. Once the meat is nearly done, add the coconut cream and vinegar. Adjust the seasoning if needed.

Nutrition Information

Calories per serving: 381

Carbohydrates: 2 g

Protein: 27.9 g

Fat: 24.5 g

Sugar: 0 g

Sodium: 0 mg

Fiber: 0.9 g

16. Spaghetti Squash with Shrimp Scampi

Prep time: 30 minutes

Serves: 4

Ingredients

- 2 cups chicken broth
- 1 small onion, chopped
- 2 1/2 teaspoon lemon-garlic seasoning

- 1 tablespoon butter or ghee
- 3 pounds spaghetti squash, cut crosswise and seeds removed
- 3/4 pounds shrimp, shelled and deveined
- salt and pepper to taste

Instructions

1. Pour broth in the Crock-Pot and stir in the lemon-garlic seasoning, onion, and butter.
2. Take the spaghetti squash and cook on high for hours.
3. Once cooked, remove the spaghetti squash from the Crock-Pot and run a fork through the meat to create the strands.
4. Take the squash strands back to the Crock-Pot and add the shrimps.
5. Season with salt and pepper.
6. Continue cooking on high for 30 minutes or until the shrimps have turned pink.

Nutrition Information

Calories per serving: 363.3

Carbohydrates: 1 g

Protein: 33 g

Fat: 21.2 g

Sugar: 0 g

Sodium: 276.2 mg

Fiber: 0.1 g

17. Crock-Pot Garlic and Shrimps

Prep time: 20 minutes

Serves: 10

Ingredients

- 3/4 cup extra-virgin olive oil
- 6 cloves of garlic, sliced
- 1 teaspoon smoked Spanish paprika
- 1 teaspoon salt

- 1/4 teaspoon black pepper
- 1/4 teaspoon red pepper flakes, crushed
- 2 pounds raw shrimp, shells removed and deveined
- 1 tablespoon parsley, minced

Instructions

1. In a small bowl, mix together olive oil, garlic, paprika, salt, pepper, and red pepper flakes.
2. Take the shrimp in the Crock-Pot and pour the spice mixture.
3. Stir to mix all ingredients.
4. Cook on low for 1 hour.
5. Garnish with parsley.

Nutrition Information

Calories per serving: 429

Carbohydrates: 1 g

Protein: 18 g

Fat: 24.5 g

Sugar: 0 g

Sodium: 211 mg

Fiber: 0 g

18. Pork Stew with Oyster Mushrooms

Prep time: 25 minutes

Serves: 4

Ingredients

- 2 tablespoon coconut oil
- 1 medium onion, chopped
- 1 clove of garlic, chopped
- 2 pounds pork loin, cut into cubes
- salt and pepper to taste
- 2 tablespoons oregano
- 2 tablespoons dried mustard
- 1/2 teaspoon ground nutmeg

- 1 1/2 cups bone broth
- 2 pounds oyster mushroom, rinsed
- 1/4 cup full-fat coconut milk
- 1/4 cup ghee
- 3 tablespoon capers

Instructions

1. In a skillet, melt the coconut oil over medium flame. Sauté the onion and garlic until fragrant. Add the pork loin and brown all sides. Season with salt and pepper to taste.
2. Transfer the sautéed meat, garlic, and onions in the Crock-Pot.
3. Add the oregano, mustard, nutmeg, bone broth, and oyster mushrooms.
4. Give a stir and cook on low for 10 hours.
5. Before the meat is nearly cooked, add the coconut milk and ghee.
6. Once done cooking, garnish with capers.

Nutrition Information

Calories per serving: 734

Carbohydrates: 12.5 g

Protein: 50.4 g

Fat: 48.9 g

Sugar: 2.3 g

Sodium: 1118 mg

Fiber: 7.9 g

19. Easy Crock-Pot Pork Loin

Prep time: 40 minutes

Serves: 12

Ingredients

- 5 pounds pork loin
- salt and pepper to taste
- 2 onions, chopped

- 3 cups beef broth

Instructions

1. Season the pork loin with salt and pepper.
2. Take inside the Crock-Pot and arrange the onions around the roast.
3. Pour the beef broth.
4. Cook on low for 10 hours until tender.

Nutrition Information

Calories per serving: 372

Carbohydrates: 0 g

Protein: 37.5 g

Fat: 23.4 g

Sugar: 0 g

Sodium: 261 mg

Fiber: 0 g

20. Sticky Chicken Wings

Prep time: 20 minutes

Serves: 6

Ingredients

- 3 tablespoons coconut aminos
- 2 tablespoons garlic, minced
- 1 tablespoon ginger, minced
- 1 teaspoon sesame oil
- 1/4 teaspoon salt
- 1 tablespoon xanthan gum
- 3 pounds chicken wings
- 2 tablespoons Chinese five-spice powder
- 3/4 teaspoon red pepper flakes
- Toasted sesame seeds for garnish

Instructions

1. Mix all ingredients except the sesame seeds.

2. Stir to coat the chicken wings.
3. Cook on low for 6 hours.
4. Garnish with sesame seeds.

Nutrition Information

Calories per serving: 475

Carbohydrates: 3 g

Protein: 31.8 g

Fat: 21 g

Sugar: 0 g

Sodium: 274 mg

Fiber: 0.9 g

21. Chicken and Kale Tortilla Stew

Prep time: 55 minutes

Serves: 6

Ingredients

- 4 cups of kale, stems removed and chopped
- 6 cups chicken broth
- 2 large chicken breasts
- 1 can crushed tomatoes
- 1 can sweetcorn
- 1/4 cup lime juice, freshly squeezed
- 1 can green chilies
- 2 tablespoons minced garlic
- 1 teaspoon cumin powder
- 2 tablespoons chili powder
- 1 teaspoon paprika
- 2 teaspoons garlic powder
- 1/4 cup Greek yogurt

Instructions

1. Take all ingredients except the Greek yogurt in the Crock-Pot.
2. Give a stir to mix all ingredients.

3. Cook on low for 5 hours.
4. Add the Greek yogurt and continue cooking on high for another hour.

Nutrition Information

Calories per serving: 362

Carbohydrates: 10 g

Protein: 25 g

Fat: 10 g

Sugar: 1.5 g

Sodium: 159 mg

Fiber: 6.3 g

22. Italian Chicken with Zucchini Noodles

Prep time: 1 hour and 10 minutes

Serves: 6

Ingredients

- 1/2 cup chicken broth
- 1 teaspoon Italian seasoning
- 4 teaspoons tomato paste
- 1 pound chicken breast
- 2 tomatoes, chopped
- 1 1/2 cups asparagus
- 1 cup snap peas, halved
- salt and pepper to taste
- 4 zucchini noodles, cut into noodle-like strips
- 1 cup commercial pesto
- Parmesan cheese for garnish
- Basil for garnish

Instructions

1. Take the chicken broth, Italian seasoning, tomato paste, chicken breasts, tomatoes, asparagus, and peas in the Crock-Pot. Give a swirl and season with salt and pepper to taste.

2. Close the lid and cook on low for 6 hours. Let it cool before assembling.
3. Assemble the noodles by placing the chicken mixture on top of the zucchini noodles. Add commercial pesto and garnish with Parmesan cheese and basil leaves.

Nutrition Information

Calories per serving: 429.7

Carbohydrates: 6 g

Protein: 32 g

Fat: 26 g

Sugar: 0.4 g

Sodium: 0 mg

Fiber: 4.2 g

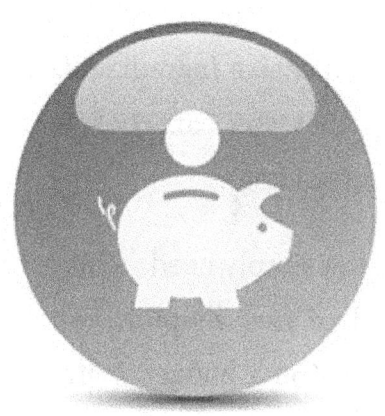

Chapter 6: Keto Meal Prep on a Budget

As much as there is a perception out there that the ketogenic diet is expensive, it isn't really true. It is possible to be on a keto diet comfortably on a budget. We shall learn in this chapter how to do keto meal prep on a budget of $50 weekly or even less.

The truth is, there are expensive ingredients for some recipes that can make it an expensive affair. The classic low-carb keto foods, like meat, leafy vegetables, and high-fat fish can be expensive. However, for every one of the expensive ingredients, there are high-quality alternatives and substitutes that you can cook with that keep in mind the nutritional requirements of keto.

Keto on a diet simply needs a bit of ingenuity and planning to get it done. By the end of this chapter, you will know how to eat a high-quality ketogenic diet on a budget. With some of the money-saving tips already discussed and the insights you will get here, you should hack the keto diet on a budget.

There are so many tricks available to you, like buying supplies in bulk, looking for deals and discounts, and shopping at farm markets, which guarantee you savings and will easily support you if you are on a budget.

The benefits of keto diet on a budget:

- You will be able to stay on the diet despite low finances.
- There are still high-quality recipe alternatives and substitutes.
- Saves you money.
- You will still get the required calories and macros.
- You do not have to strain financially.
- No stress from lack of money to by the high-priced recipe items.

6.1 How to Succeed on a $50-a-Week Keto Meal Prep Plan

Here are some great ideas to help you to achieve a keto meal prep on $50 for a week of keto meals:

- **Plan in advance.**

Apart from keeping your meal plan simple, this is the most important point for cost-saving. Planning will save you money through the whole process—from purchase to restocking.

Planning prevents impulse and unnecessary purchases because you will have to shop as per a predetermined list.

- **Opt for cheaper ingredient alternatives or substitutes.**

Always go for cheaper recipe alternatives to the more expensive seasonal or classic recipe ingredients. There are high-priced and low-priced items for each food or ingredient category.

- *Cheese*

    This is a staple of the keto diet. Avoid specialty cheeses and buy a block of regular cheese and grate or shred it yourself.

- *Fish*

    Fish is a high-quality and healthy keto fat and protein source but is often expensive. Use canned fish in place of fresh fish if you are on a diet.

- *Poultry*

    If you have to buy chicken in parts, go for the cheaper cuts like thighs, legs, and wings. Alternatively, buy a whole chicken which is cheaper than buying parts.

- *Meat*

    Go for fatty meat cuts. They are cheaper than lean cuts, and buy from a butchery rather than a supermarket.

- *Vegetables*

    Vegetables are integral to the success of the keto diet. Buy frozen vegetables instead of fresh low-carb vegetables, which are usually expensive at supermarkets. Frozen vegetables are cheap and do not go bad as fast as fresh vegetables.

- *Eggs*

    Stock a lot of eggs in your pantry. They are one of the cheaper protein sources and are versatile for keto recipes.

- **Shop in bulk.**

There is no better way of saving money or working within a budget that shopping for ingredients in bulk because it is cheaper. Stock up items on sale every time you come across them.

- **Be on the lookout for price discounts and offer.**

If you are on a budget, be on the lookout for price reductions and deals on quantities. This is a great way of getting more for less.

- **Avoid impulse buying.**

Simply put, do not purchase anything that you do not have on your shopping list; otherwise, you will mess up your budget.

- **Buy items online.**

Items are generally cheaper online. Take advantage of online stores to save money and get more items for at your weekly budget. You will be amazed at how much you save and get by buying things online than at the local supermarket.

- **Keep your meal prep simple.**

The simpler your keto meal plan is, the cheaper and easier it will be on your finances.

Tip: Do not buy a product or ingredient you have never used before in bulk because it may not be what you like or want. Buy a little to try and only buy in bulk if it is something for you.

Quick Start Action Step

Sticking to a keto diet on a $50-per-week meal plan is possible. You can even spend less depending on your preferences and meals choices. Use the insights in this chapter and take the simple options above to keep you healthy on keto when you are on a budget.

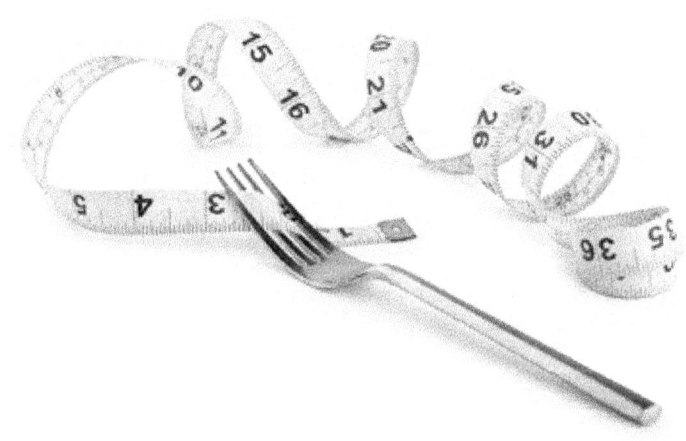

Chapter 7: Keto Meal Prep for Weight Loss

Just as you can do keto meal planning on a lean weekly budget, you can do the same for weight loss. A tight budget cannot prevent you from getting ingredients focused on weight loss.

As you are now aware, the ketogenic diet can be used for putting on weight, for maintaining the weight you are at, or for losing weight. For each of the three options, there are different and specific keto calories and macros that are effective and recommended for desired results.

Fat burning for weight loss is one of the main benefits of ketosis and is probably the reason why it is so popular. Keto makes people feel great and more satiated, which helps you to eat less of what you should not eat. It elevates mental and physical energy, which should not be impeded by low finances.

Achieving weight loss through keto on a lean budget is possible, and you should still be able to buy the weight-loss ingredients within your budget. Much of it is similar to what we have discussed in the previous chapter but directed at keto items for weight loss.

There are many keto weight-loss recipes and ingredients that can be cooked and bought respectively without spending so much money. Since dieting is about nutrition content in an ingredient of food, you will find nutrient-rich foods that are not necessarily in the high-price bracket. Make your pick from the list of affordable keto weight-loss ingredients further down.

7.1 Benefits of Keto Meal Pep for Weight Loss

The following are the foremost benefits of keto meal planning for weight loss:

- It elevates mental focus and concentration.
- It is highly effective at burning fat.
- It infuses your body and muscles with energy.
- It curtails constant hunger pangs.
- It helps in blood sugar balance and regulation.
- It improves skin health and fights acne.
- It controls cholesterol and triglyceride levels.
- It improves hormonal regulation in women, especially for severe PMS symptoms.

7.2 Affordable Weight-Loss Ingredients for Keto Meal Prep on a Budget

The following are great affordable keto weight-loss ingredients for one on a budget:

1. *Avocado*

Avocado is a ketogenic diet essential for healthy fat content, minerals, and vitamins. Not only is it good for its rich fat content but it also helps keto beginners to deal with symptoms of keto flu. It is high in fat and very low on carbs.

2. *Kimchi and sauerkraut*

Fermented foods carrying good bacteria, and prebiotic fibers are good for gut health. Studies have found that a healthy bacteria balance in your stomach can help to reduce fat mass.

3. *Eggs*

Eggs are the most versatile keto foods and one of the healthiest proteins for weight loss. Eggs will leave you feeling full and will keep you from packing extra calories.

4. *Garlic*

Garlic, as you know, has many long-exploited health benefits. A study found that garlic can help with weight loss.

5. *Leafy vegetables*

Collard greens, kale, spinach, and Swiss chard are great and affordable keto weight-loss foods. They are high in fiber, which slows digestion and iron nutrients which helps the body absorb the nutrients efficiently.

6. *Nuts*

Nuts are high in healthy fat and are not fattening as you may think. Look for recipes that incorporate them. Nuts improve metabolism and help with weight loss because of the high fiber content, which leaves you with a feeling of being full, thus keeping you from eating. Here are the best nuts:

- Almonds (carbs: 6 grams)
- Brazil nuts (carbs: 3 grams)

- Cashews (carbs: 9 grams)
- Macadamia nuts (carbs: 4 grams)
- Pecans (carbs: 4 grams)
- Pistachios (carbs: 8 grams)
- Walnuts (carbs: 4 grams)

7. *Protein powder*

Use protein powder to complement and supplement protein in your meals. Get protein benefits without extra calories—no extra fat or carbohydrates.

8. *Vinegar*

Use vinegar to replace high-calorie additions or condiments to your food.

9. *Pasture-raised chicken*

Eat free-range chicken and benefit from the fat-loss benefits of protein.

10. *Cruciferous vegetables*

Vegetables such as broccoli and cauliflower fall in this group and are keto staples because of their weight-loss benefits. They are a source of sulforaphane and fiber. Sulforaphane has been linked with stimulating energy-burning brown fat and improving gut health. It is also linked to fighting obesity.

11. *Olives and olive oil*

Olive oil helps with fat loss and promotes a leaner body. The healthy fats in olive oil and its anti-inflammatory properties are key to weight loss.

12. *Chilies*

Chilies have fat-burning properties, which are why obesity is low among people who consume a lot of chilies. Chilies contain capsaicin, which reduces appetite and boosts the burning of body fat.

13. *Coconut oil*

Coconut oil has healthy fats and promotes fat loss. A study of obese men found that supplementing their diet with two tablespoons (30 mL) of coconut oil daily helped them cut their waistlines by one inch.

These are some of the top keto ingredients that you can get easily when you are working with a tight grocery budget to help you with keto meal prep for weight loss.

Quick Start Action Step

Pick some of these keto ingredients to help you make the most out of your keto meal prep for weight loss.

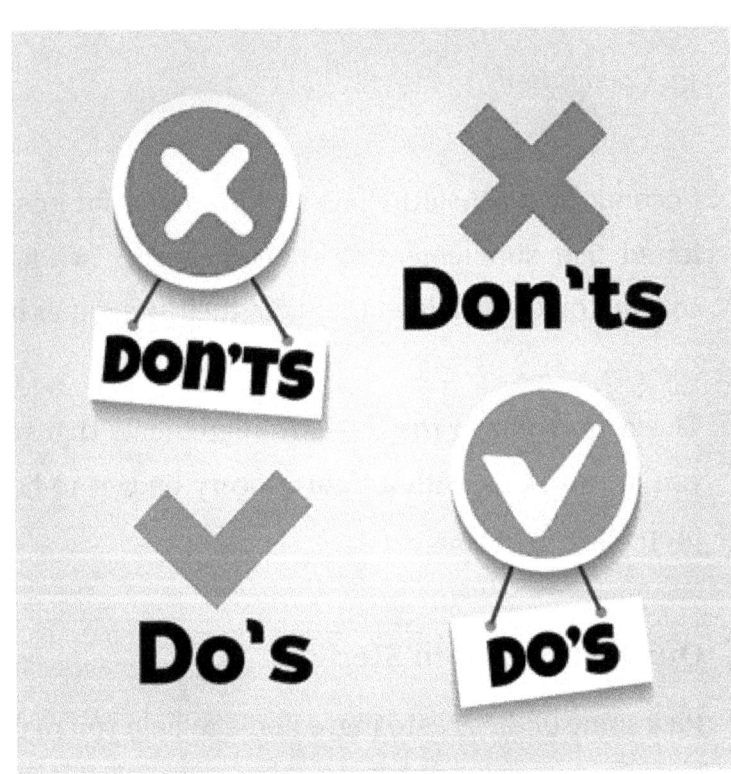

Chapter 8: Keto Meal Prep—Mistakes to Avoid

There are some common mistakes that people make on the keto diet that should be avoided because you will never succeed if you keep them up. In fact, it is possible to make some of these mistakes without knowing it. Keto meal prep is really effective if you stick to the script.

Keto does not have to drain your wallet. Doing things the correct way will help you see great returns on investment. Planning and preparation are key to making keto meal prepping very easy, and it ensures success.

8.1 Common Keto Mistakes

The following are some of the common keto meal prep mistakes you want to avoid:

1. Lack of Proper Planning

We already discussed the importance of planning for keto meal prepping. Lack of planning means that you open the doors for many things to go wrong. Failing to prepare means you should prepare to fail.

If you do not plan, you will eat the wrong things, waste time, and lose value for your money. An essential part of planning is doing extensive research into the ingredients and recipes you want to cook.

2. Eating Too Much Protein

You know the macro ratios required for successful ketosis. Eating too much protein is very easy and is a common mistake that must be suppressed. Too much protein consumption leads to elevated blood sugar because it is converted into glucose and defeating ketosis.

3. Low Mineral Intake

Ketosis increases acid production in the body, which lowers the body pH. Basic food minerals help balance out this state and create a normal pH.

4. Not Eating Enough Fat

Keto relies on fat for body energy; if you do not eat enough, you are putting a strain on the body, especially because you have cut on the other energy sources of the body.

5. Tracking on Carbohydrate Intake

Many people quickly forget that they should be tracking everything they eat and only track carb macros in the endeavor to reduce the carbs they consume. When you track only one macro, it is very easy to overeat another.

6. Eating Too Much Unhealthy Fat

As much as the keto diet is high-fat, consumption of too much of the wrong fats is wrong. Eating too much unsaturated fat should be avoided.

7. Not Drinking Enough Water

It is very easy not to drink enough water, and this is a common mistake by many people, especially newbies to the keto diet. Water is a must for keeping your body healthy while on the journey to ketosis and to maintain it. Dehydration while on ketosis can lead to kidney problems or failure. Put water at the top of your list.

8. Eating Only Animal Products

The efficacy of the keto diet can be misleading if you are not well informed. Include all food types, especially healthy vegetables. Plant foods are important sources of phytonutrients, vitamins, and fiber.

9. Eating Too Much Dairy Products

Consume dairy in moderation of on a keto diet. Dairy products are high in calories, which is counterproductive to what you want. You should burn more calories than you consume.

Forgetting physical exercise

Do not forget as much as the keto diet if efficient at burning fat. Exercise is important while on a ketosis diet to stimulate muscle building and calories and fat burning.

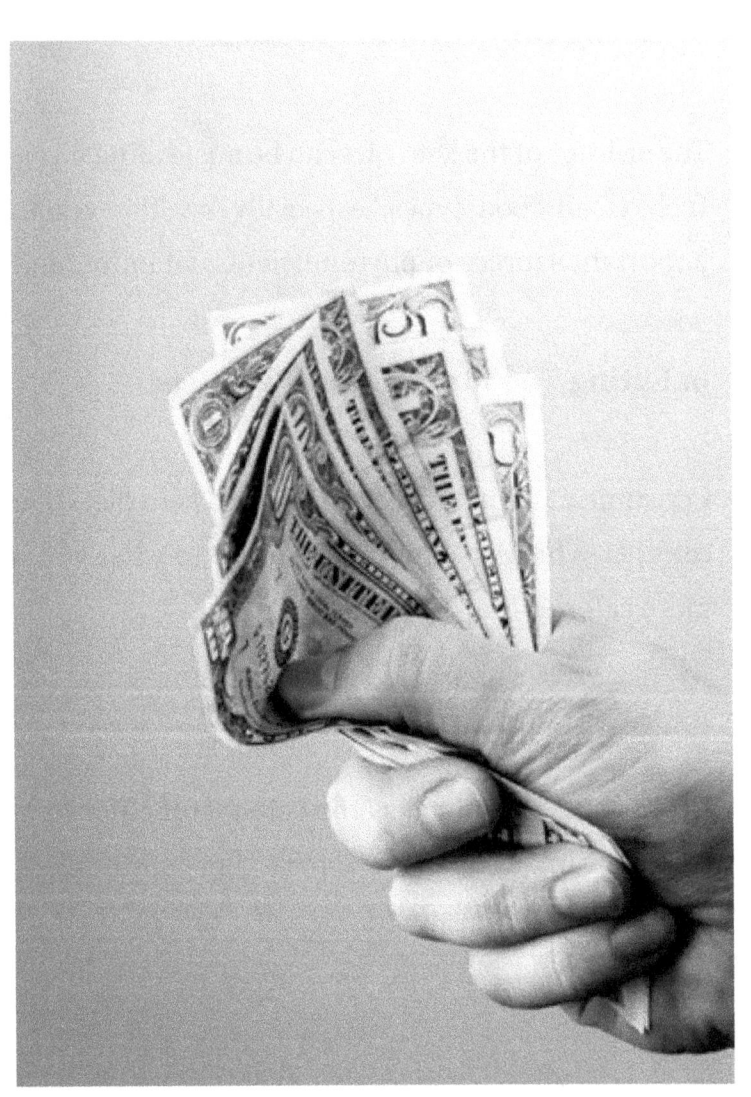

Bonus Chapter: Money-Savings Tips When Shopping

Here is a summary of keto meal planning money-saving tips when you go shopping:

- Much like shopping for everything else, making use of sales. Special discounts and coupons will save you a lot of cash.
- Buy items in bulk, enough for every week's meal prep; they will be cheaper. Also, refrigerate and freeze items just long enough to use.
- If you can, grow some of the vegetables you use on your own. It is much healthier and, of course, cheaper.
- Go for seasonal produce (fruits and vegetable) because they are cheaper and are more likely to be on sale.
- Shop at the farmers market for dairy, fruits, meats, and vegetables.
- Always go for fresh products. Avoid packaged produce because of the extra expense you will incur.
- Keep your meal plan simple. The fewer the ingredients you require for your meals, the less money you will need to buy them.
- Go for frozen vegetables when fresh options are not available.
- Always buy a whole chicken and cut it yourself. Buying cuts is expensive.
- Make most purchases when there are price deals, such as discounts and clearance sales.
- Shopping online is cheaper.

Measurement Conversions

Liquid Volumes		
mL	US	fl. oz.
5	1 tsp.	
15	1 tbsp.	1/2
30	1/8 c.	1
60	1/4 c.	2
78	1/3 c.	
118	1/2 c.	4
158	2/3 c.	
177	3/4 c.	6
237	1 c.	8
355	1 1/2 c.	12
474	2 c.	16
710	3 c.	24
946	4 c.	32

When exact measures aren't necessary, you can round 1 c = 250 mL.

Dry Weights	
Grams	Ounce to Pounds
28	1
57	2
85	3

113	4 oz. = 1/4 lb.
151	1/3 lbs.
227	8 oz. = 1/2 lb.
302	2/3 lb.
340	12 oz. = 3/4 lb.
454	1 lb.
907	2 lbs.

Oven Temperatures	
Celsius	**Fahrenheit**
140°	285°
150°	300°
160°	320°
170°	338°
180°	356°
200°	392°
220°	425°
225°	437°

Conclusion

Thank you again for owning this book!

I hope this book was able to help you to help you understand how to do keto meal planning successfully. We defined what keto meal prepping and planning is and delved into the benefits of adapting meal planning for the keto diet.

Further, we looked at the steps required of proper meal planning and went through what you need to do from start to finish. By now, I am confident that you know the essentials of keto meal prepping for your pantry and kitchen. You know how to shop and the right containers to store your food for the week.

We did not stop there, we looked at the importance of macros for keto meal planning and got insights on how to calculate macros and why we should.

This book has dedicated two chapters to keto recipes. Chapter 4 carries simple and easy go-to keto recipes for keto meal plan beginners while the next chapter is a reservoir of great keto meals that will keep you excited about meal planning for months.

More importantly, chapters 6 and 7 look at how to shop for keto ingredients on a budget, which is important because a lean budget should not hinder us from achieving and maintaining ketosis.

The next step is for you to take the insights and tips from this book and ingratiate them into your keto meal prep plan. The benefits are numerous, and the joy you will get from the information and the recipes in this book is invaluable.

Thank you and good luck!

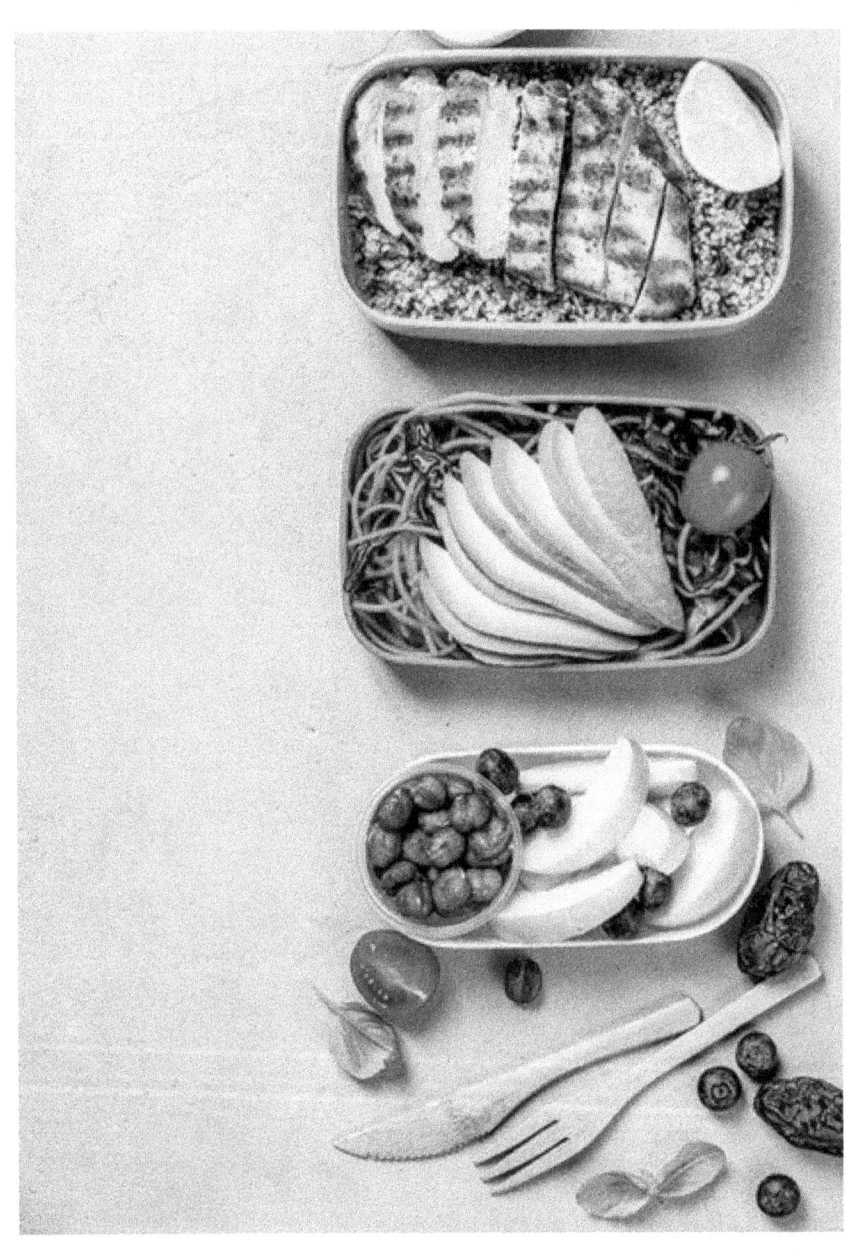

Intermittent Fasting for Beginners

Simple and Easy-to-Follow Weight Loss Guide on How to Lose Weight Faster, Feel Better and Live a Healthy Lifestyle

Jason Brad Stephens

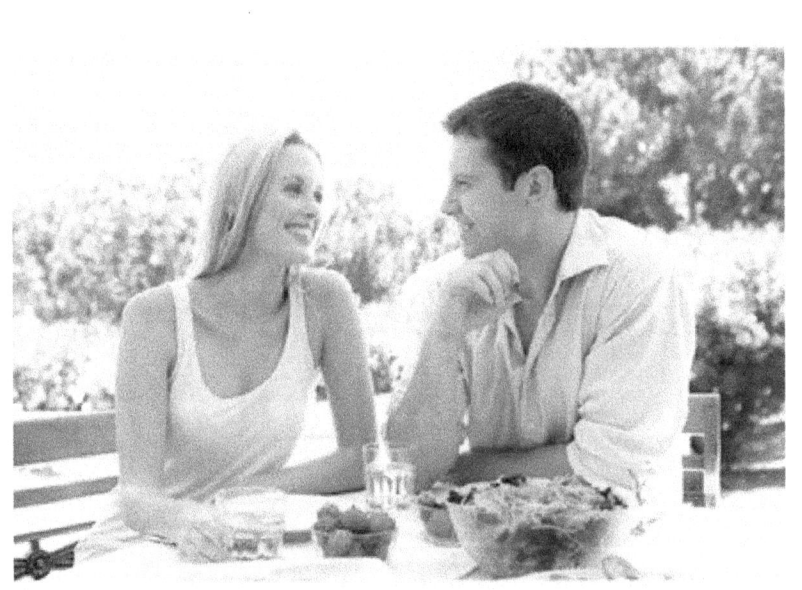

Table of Contents

Introduction

Chapter 1: Getting Started with Intermittent Fasting

Chapter 2: Dealing with Overweight Dilemma

Chapter 3: The Problem with our Diet

Chapter 4: Intermittent Fasting: An Overview on How to Lose Weight Faster

Chapter 5: Intermittent Fasting: Best Foods to Eat

Chapter 6: Intermittent Fasting: Best Time to Eat in a Day

Chapter 7: Picking the Right Meal Plan

Chapter 8: The One Meal a Day approach

Chapter 9: Healthy Recipes

Chapter 10: Mistakes to Avoid and Who Should Not Fast

Chapter 11: When You Are Not Seeing Results

Chapter 12: Living the Healthy, Guilt-Free Lifestyle

Bonus Chapter: Benefits with Ketogenic Diet

Conclusion

Introduction:

According to a study that was conducted by the World Health Organization, it was revealed that in 2016, more than 1.9 billion adults, aged above 18 years from across the globe, were overweight. 39% of adults aged above 18 years were overweight and 13% were obese in 2016. Worse still, 41 million children aged below 5 years were either overweight, or obese.

Nonetheless, all hope is not lost, as the problem of obesity is preventable. Today, we are experiencing a fitness revolution in many parts of the world as people are becoming more aware of the dangers that a sedentary lifestyle poses to human health. People are taking up fitness, yoga, rhumba, and even Zumba classes, hoping to shed a couple of kilos and to tone their bodies.

However, one important point that many people fail to understand is that weight loss is a three-part process that involves fitness and physical activity, a positive mindset and, most importantly, diet. Your diet, both the quality and quantity, is very important in your weight loss program. It will determine how fast you lose weight, and if you will regain the weight that you have lost.

While there are many factors that cause obesity, it is scientifically proven that obesity is hormonal, and not a result of calorie imbalance or excessive consumption of calories. When we eat, the food is broken down and converted into glucose, which is a source of energy for the body. Insulin is a hormone that is involved in the absorption of glucose, and the storage of excess glucose as fats. Hence, it causes cells in the body to absorb this glucose for energy. However, when we eat excessively, the insulin in the bloodstream increases, signaling the body to store most of this glucose as fat, contributing to obesity.

Having seen that insulin is responsible for most cases of obesity, the natural solution is to find ways that will reduce the amount of insulin in the bloodstream. Two of the most common ways of reducing insulin levels in the bloodstream are: the ketogenic diet, and the intermittent fasting diet.

Intermittent fasting is characterized by distinct periods of eating and fasting. It is an important tool that involves calorie restriction, alternating between regular feeding days and fasting days, or limiting the number of hours that you get to eat within the day. There are different methods of intermittent fasting, each with its own distinct characteristics and dietary requirements. They include: the popular 16/8 (which has different variants), the eat-stop-eat method, the 5:2 method, the 4:3 method, and meal skipping, amongst others.

According to Jimmy Moore, fasting is not just any other "F-word". It is a method that dates back to the times of the ancient Greeks and the Egyptians that has proven itself time and time again. Many people who hear the word "fasting" believe that it is synonymous with starvation. However, this book will take you through the fundamental differences between these two concepts and explain to you just why intermittent fasting could be the saving grace of all humanity.

One of the main reasons why intermittent fasting has quickly risen in popularity is that it not only allows you to lose weight, but also improves your health and general well-being. The diet has been associated with increased metabolism, reduced insulin resistance, reduced inflammation, retarded growth of cancer cells, a reduced risk of developing heart diseases, anti-aging and, of course, weight loss.

The diet calls for highly nutritious foods and recipes which should contain both the macro and micronutrients. The meals should be high in proteins, healthy fats, and oils, but low in carbohydrates. This allows the body to remain in a state of ketosis where it burns down the fat reserves for energy, instead of relying on glucose from carbohydrates. Proteins are particularly important, as they nourish the muscles and the body's organs, while creating a feeling of satiation. This reduces hunger pangs and cravings. Some of the foods that are strictly forbidden in this diet include: white foods, fatty cuts of beef and pork, carbonated drinks, and all foods that are rich in starches and simple sugars.

It is arguable that the most important aspect of the intermittent fasting diet is developing the discipline and willpower to stick to the diet, despite the cravings and hunger pangs that people experience. This is because hunger is a powerful feeling that can demotivate and disorient you.

Many people cite that the most difficult aspect of the diet is not the hunger that you experience, but instead is the sheer determination that it will take for you to overcome the conventional three-meals-a-day habit.

The main reason why the intermittent fasting diet fails is because people give in to their bodily urges and social demands in relation to food. Inconsistency, and the inability to follow through with your caloric restrictions, will set you up for failure.

Due to the extreme nature of the intermittent fasting diet, it is not recommended for all people. If you are known to have a history of an eating disorder, or are underweight, this diet may not be for you. Pregnant and lactating women too should avoid this diet. All women should carefully approach this diet as there are instances where it interferes with the natural menstrual cycle. People who suffer from type 2 diabetes, or any other medical conditions, should also approach the diet with caution. Generally, it is highly recommended that you seek the advice of a medical practitioner before starting the diet.

In this book, we aim to provide conclusive knowledge of the intermittent fasting diet, while clarifying some of the myths and misconceptions that are often related to this topic. As a bonus, we will also analyze the ketogenic diet, clearly highlighting why the two diets are the most effective in weight loss.

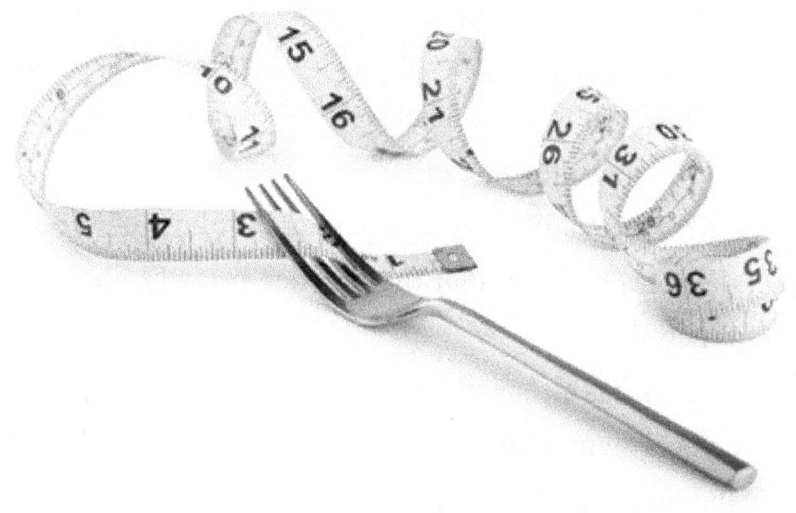

Chapter 1: Getting Started with Intermittent Fasting

1.1 Fasting: Definition and a Brief History

Many people use the word fasting interchangeably with the word starvation. People who use a fasting diet to lose weight will claim, jokingly, that they are starving themselves to lose weight. In such a situation, the correct terminology is fasting, and not starving.

Fasting is fundamentally different from starvation in one way: the ability to exercise control. Starvation refers to the involuntary abstention from eating. Starving people have no idea where, or when, they will have their next meal. Their failure to eat is neither deliberate, nor controlled. Fasting is the *voluntary* abstention from eating. When fasting, food is readily available, but you deliberately choose not to eat it. It is usually done for spiritual, health, and other reasons.

The concept of fasting dates to the days of the ancient Greeks when devotees believed that the practice brought about physical and spiritual renewal.

Fasting has also played a major role in some religions, where it is believed to be a sign of penitence and self-control. In Islam, Muslims fast during the holy month of Ramadhan. The Roman Catholics observe the 40-day fast during the Lenten season. In Judaism, the Day of Atonement is marked as an annual fast day.

Modified fasting, also known as intermittent fasting, is a dietary pattern that involves cycles of eating and fasting. There are different methods of going about intermittent fasting. They include: the 16/8 method, the eat-stop-eat method, the 5:2 diet, and the 4:3 diet. However, the underlying principle is that all these methods split either the day or the week into distinct periods of eating and fasting.

Limiting food intake to the middle of the day, which is a form of intermittent fasting, decreases body weight and fat, glucose and insulin levels, insulin resistance, and inflammation. This leads to mild calorie restriction without necessarily counting calories. Consistency in intermittent fasting is therefore very important for one to lose weight. It is more of a lifestyle than it is a short-term diet.

While intermittent fasting is a conscious effort to skip meals, or to exclusively eat at certain times of the day, regular fasting involves abstaining from food for longer durations of time, mostly days.

While fasting, the calorie intake is usually zero. The body shifts to a state of ketosis where any stored body fat is burned to produce ketones for energy. Fasting may seem to be the quicker way to lose excess weight. It can be detrimental in the long run because it depletes all the glycogen stored in the liver, and the body could begin breaking down its own muscles and organs for energy.

1.2 Benefits of Intermittent Fasting

In the past, humans engaged in food-seeking which would last anywhere from a couple of hours to a few days. The mechanisms that allowed humans to survive such periods of fasting are believed to have numerous benefits, which have been negated by the present-day sedentary lifestyle characterized by continuous and abundant food supply.

Based on a scientific study by, intermittent fasting could lead to:

- An extended lifespan. Intermittent fasting diets are believed to alter the mitochondrial networks inside the energy producing cells, increasing lifespan and promoting good health.
- Protection from obesity, cardiovascular disease, diabetes, and hypertension. During intermittent fasting, the insulin levels in the blood drop significantly, facilitating fat burning. The drop in insulin consequently leads to a drop in blood sugar levels, which decreases the risk of type 2 diabetes. A drop in insulin levels also leads to an increase in the breakdown of body fat, facilitating the

use of fat as an energy source. This greatly reduces the cholesterol levels in the body, and cases of obesity and cardiovascular diseases.

- Improvement in insulin sensitivity. As a result of the decreased insulin levels in the bloodstream, the cells become more sensitive to any insulin released into the bloodstream. As such, it does not accumulate within the blood.
- Retarded growth of tumors. Periodic fasting leads to a decrease in the growth of cancerous tumors and increased sensitivity to chemotherapy. When cancerous cells are exposed to environments that contain lower glucose levels, proliferation and cell death quickly follow. This is a process known as cell starvation.
- Reduced inflammation. Inflammation is a common symptom of all chronic diseases that we face today. It is known to occur whenever the body is trying to heal itself. However, whenever inflammation occurs for too long, it is associated with some negative effects.
- An intermittent fasting diet involves increased consumption of foods that are rich in fats and oils. These high fats and oils decrease the production of Leukotriene B4 (LTB4) which is involved in various cellular processes that are related to inflammation.
- Enhanced brain functionality. In addition, through intermittent fasting, we have a significant decrease in inflammatory markers such as cytokines and C-reactive protein.
- Improved brain functionality and cognitive functions. Intermittent fasting, just like exercising, leads to the production of a protein called brain-derived neurotrophic factor (BDNF) within the nerve cells. This protein is especially important in learning, memory, and in the production of new nerve cells in the hippocampus.

Other benefits of intermittent fasting include: improving the circulation of cholesterol and triglycerides, resistance to ischemic injury, improved survival from myocardial ischemia, efficient metabolism, and reduced oxidative stress. Hence, we see that intermittent fasting is an effective and convenient lifestyle habit that will make your life simpler, while also improving your health.

1.3 Types of Intermittent Fasting

Intermittent fasting has grown in popularity as one of the recommended ways to lose weight while improving your health and general well-being. Some of the popular methods are:

1. The 16/8 method:

    This is believed to be the most popular method, owing to its sustainability and ease of application. It involves restricting the consumption of foods and calorie-containing beverages to eight hours per day and abstaining from food for the remaining 16 hours. For example, one may decide to eat food between noon and 8 PM only.

    During the 8-hour eating period, one should focus on eating healthy meals and drinking calorie-free drinks such as water and unsweetened teas and coffee.

    However, the windows may vary from one person to the next, with some people preferring to eat within a 6 hour window (18/6), and others preferring to eat over a 4 hour window (20/4). Nonetheless, the method is easy to follow and provides results with minimal effort.

2. Eat-stop-eat:

    This is a form of intermittent fasting that was put together by Brad Pilon. It involves fasting for 24-hour periods either once or twice a week. On the other five or six days, one should concentrate on eating responsibly while keeping the overall calorie intake with the desired range.

    The fast can begin either at breakfast, lunch, or dinner, as long as an individual fasts for 24 consecutive hours. During your fasting days, you must make sure to take in as few calories as possible. It is recommended that you should only drink plain or sparkling water, unsweetened tea or coffee, and diet soda. It is important to note that you should break your fast with a regularly sized meal. Avoid compensating for the fast by feasting on a large meal.

3. The 5:2 diet:

It is also known as the fast diet and is currently the most popular intermittent fasting diet. The diet involves 5 normal eating days and 2 days in which calorie intake is restricted to 500-600 calories per day, or to 25% of your daily calorie intake.

The choice of eating and fasting days is entirely at your discretion, as long as there is a non-fasting day between any two consecutive fasting days. During normal eating days, you should stick to healthy foods and calorie-free drinks, or else you will not lose any weight at all.

This diet is easier to stick to, as opposed to traditional calorie-restricted diets.

4. The 4:3 diet:

Also known as the alternate day fasting, this involves a normal eating day followed by a fasting day. This method, though effective for weight loss, is an extreme form of intermittent fasting and is not suitable for beginners or people with different health conditions. In addition, it may be difficult to maintain this kind of diet long-term. On the normal days, you are advised to eat as much you want. On the fasting days, you are advised to eat a 400-calorie meal and a 100-calorie snack, to drink lots of water, tea and coffee, and to chew sugarless gum. However, some people recommend completely avoiding solid foods on fasting days.

5. Meal Skipping

This is a method that is especially common among beginners. It involves skipping specific meals of the day depending on your level of hunger or time constraints. In addition, the meals consumed must be healthy to ensure the success of the diet.

The diet plan is especially successful when you keep track and respond moderately to your hunger needs. This implies that you only eat food when you are hungry and otherwise avoid any food.

6. The Warrior Diet

    This is an extreme form of intermittent fasting diet that was developed in 2001 by Ori Hofmekler. The diet involves eating small portions of raw fruits and vegetables during a 20-hour fasting period and eating one large meal at night during a 4-hour eating period. It can therefore be described as a cycle of fasting and overeating.

    During the 20-hour fasting period, you should consume small amounts of dairy products, hard-boiled eggs, raw fruits and vegetables, and calorie-free fluids. On the other hand, during the 4-hour eating period, you should consume plenty of fruits, vegetables, proteins, and healthy fats. Carbohydrates should also be consumed, though in fewer quantities.

    The diet is based on the fact that humans are nocturnal eaters and absorb nutrients at night in line with the circadian rhythms. It is mainly used by individuals who have tried other intermittent fasting diets. Beginners should therefore proceed with caution.

Your Quick Start Action Step:

Now it is your turn! Try either one of the above methods of intermittent fasting and record the results from each of the methods, identifying the one that works best for you.

It is important to note that before trying any intermittent diet, you should consult your medical practitioner for the go-ahead. Inasmuch as intermittent fasting diets are known to be beneficial in the control and management of type-2 diabetes, patients should first consult the advice of a medical practitioner.

Chapter 2: Dealing with the Overweight Dilemma

2.1 Obesity: Current Issues

Obesity refers to a condition or disorder in which excessive body fat accumulates to the extent in which it may have adverse effects on the general health of an individual. Doctors suggest that anyone with a Body Mass Index (BMI) of between 25 and 29.9 is overweight, while anyone with a BMI above 30 is obese.

According to the newly released Global Nutrition Report, obesity is a problem that costs $500 billion annually. The data shows that 63% of American women are overweight while 37% are obese.

In many developed countries such as the United States, obesity is an epidemic. The Centers for Disease Control and Prevention (CDC) estimates that in 2015–2016, 93.3 million (39.8 percent) American adults, and 13.7 million (18.5 percent) American children and teens were clinically obese.

Some of the causes of obesity are attributed to the present-day civilization that encourages indoor living and despises physical activity. They include:

- Living a sedentary lifestyle that allows for the accumulation of fats. In today's modern world, people use vehicles to move from one place to another as opposed to walking, or even cycling. Relaxation mainly involves watching movies or browsing the internet. As such, the energy generated from the food we eat is not utilized and is instead stored as fats.
- Diets that are rich in simple carbohydrates, fats, and calories. Eating large amounts of highly processed foods, fast foods, or sugary drinks leads to obesity because these foods contain high amounts of fats and calories.

- Inadequate sleep which may lead to hormonal changes which may leave you craving foods that are rich in calories. In addition, inadequate sleep leads to the secretion of signal hormones such as ghrelin, which increases appetite, and leptin, which indicates when the body is satiated. This leads to increased food intake beyond the body's requirements.
- Genetics which have an impact on the metabolism rate, and how fat is stored. Children of obese parents are more likely to be obese than children of lean parents.
- Growing older. This leads to a decreased metabolic rate and less muscle mass, making it easier to gain weight.
- Medications. Some pharmaceutical drugs lead to weight loss as a side effect. Medication for diabetes, epilepsy, and psychotics, such as anti-depressants and medicines for schizophrenia, have been known to contribute to weight gain.
- Diseases such as: polycystic ovary syndrome, insulin resistance, Cushing's syndrome, and hypothyroidism. High insulin levels lead to increased insulin resistance which implies that insulin is not absorbed by the cells in the body, but is instead stored as fat in the body, leading to obesity.
- Food addiction and aggressive marketing. Some junk and fast food producers are very aggressive in their marketing, sometimes making unhealthy food look healthy.

While the physical effects of obesity are widely documented and popularized, the psychological and emotional effects are often swept under the carpet, forgetting that patients suffering from obesity are also human.

We live in a society where slim and toned bodies are worshiped. Everything else is considered undesirable and unsightly. It then becomes easy for people suffering from obesity to suffer from anxiety and depression, and to lose their self-esteem and joy of life when society considers them to be undesirable. In extreme cases, this can lead to suicide.

However, by reading this book, you will discover that obesity is not a death sentence. You will discover the use of intermittent fasting to shed off extra kilos in a sustainable manner. This is because intermittent fasting is not merely a short-term diet that promises you instant rewards. Instead, it is a way of life that guarantees you long-term results.

2.2 Reasons Why We Can't Afford to Ignore Obesity

As mentioned earlier, obesity is an epidemic in many developed and developing countries. The problem can no longer be ignored, nor can society turn a blind eye to it, because of the large number of people who are affected by this condition.

Not only does it lead to feelings of low self-esteem and depression, but obesity also robs society of important minds and personalities through suicide. A study that was published in the American Journal of Epidemiology states that people who are morbidly obese are five times more likely to experience suicidal thoughts as opposed to those who are not.

Obesity also creates conflict in romantic relationships. Studies indicate that obese partners are likely to carry feelings of shame and embarrassment concerning their food consumption and body weight. Any criticism regarding overeating habits may lead to arguments or conflict. This situation may be worse if a partner uses derogatory language to encourage the obese partner to hit the gym.

In addition, people with obesity are more likely to suffer from serious diseases and health conditions such as: cardiovascular disease, type 2 diabetes, hypertension, stroke, gallbladder disease, and osteoporosis, amongst other diseases.

2.3 Steps on how to Approach Obesity

Losing weight is a combination of a positive mindset, healthy eating, and exercises. You cannot achieve your weight loss goals if you ignore or overindulge in one aspect in the triad.

To lose weight, an individual must first make peace with their current state and fully embrace who they are. Then, and only then, will they be able to witness real changes. In addition, you must be fully aware that losing weight will take a lot of time and effort. Most of all, you will need to make certain sacrifices and adjustments for your success.

Some of the steps you could put in place when approaching a weight loss journey are:

1. Set your goals: You will need to analyze your eating habits, current weight and any health conditions that you may have, and then create a game plan that will lead you to your goal. Inasmuch as losing weight is the ultimate goal, individuals should create smaller milestones to motivate them to move closer to that goal.

2. Surround yourself with positive energy: Avoid keeping the company of people who persistently remind you of your weight. Instead, surround yourself with people who are positive and encourage you to become your best self. For added motivation, you could join a slimming club which is a great way to meet new people who share the same goals as you.

3. Make sure your goals are realistic and attainable: Remember that the journey of a thousand miles starts with a single step. It doesn't matter how small you start, just as long as you do start. This will provide you with a platform to work towards your goal.

4. Keep a track of all your activities: You could track yourself using a food diary, an exercise log, or a spreadsheet that contains both these records. By keeping track of your fitness exercises, eating habits, and even your moods, you become more accountable to yourself and thus, even more motivated to achieve your fitness goals.

5. Avoid stepping on the scale: For many people, the scale has been associated with negative and self-destructive thoughts. To avoid getting discouraged, don't bother stepping on the scale until you are at a point where you have overcome the feelings that come with it. When at this point, make sure to weigh yourself frequently as studies show that people who weigh themselves more often are more likely to lose weight than those who do not.

6. Do not beat yourself up whenever you face minor set-backs or whenever you are unable to meet your goals. This will only serve to discourage you and will not help you to achieve your desired goal. Instead, take this set-back as an opportunity to get back on the drawing board to re-strategize.

7. Keep track of the sugars and starches in your diet: As mentioned earlier, over-consumption of foods and drinks that are rich in simple sugars and carbohydrates greatly contributes to obesity. It is therefore important to cut back on the amount of sugars and starches that you consume. In doing so, the body will have less glucose in the bloodstream and will instead burn down the fats stored in the body to produce energy. You must therefore eat mindfully to effectively deal with the problem of obesity.

8. Eat plenty of proteins, fruits, and vegetables. Ideally, you should construct your meals such that you have a high protein source, a low-carb vegetable source, and a fat source. Your intake of carbohydrates should be within the daily recommended range of 20-30 grams. High protein diets have been proven to increase metabolism and to reduce cravings and frequent snacking. The fats that you consume should be healthy, so you have no reason to be afraid of fats.

9. Focus on eating whole and unprocessed foods as opposed to white foods. This is because white foods are highly processed with most of the essential nutrients being stripped away and replaced with synthetic vitamins. Whole foods on the other hand are healthier

and more filling, reducing the occurrence of hunger pangs and cravings.

10. Drink plenty of unsweetened tea and coffee. This is because these drinks are believed to boost metabolism by 3% - 11%. In addition, they are very effective in suppressing cravings and feelings of hunger.

11. Avoid eating your foods hurriedly. People who eat very fast tend to gain more weight while those who eat slowly feel full, reducing the amount of food that they eat. In addition, eating slowly boosts the production of hormones that are known to reduce weight.

12. Take part in physical activities and exercises. This will help you to burn the calories and keep your body toned and fit. Generally, the degree of exercises varies from one person to the next. Based on age, health conditions, and weight loss goals, amongst many other factors, you could choose from low to medium to high-intensity exercises.

13. Make sure you get adequate rest. Every night, you should be able to sleep for eight hours, the daily recommended number. Poor and inadequate sleep is one of the reasons why people become obese.

Your Quick Start Action Step:

While it is universally agreed that losing weight is a difficult and sometimes a daunting task, preparation is the most critical part of the process which, when properly done, makes the whole process seem easier and less tasking.

As such, before starting your weight loss program, you should spend as much time as possible speaking to your doctor, researching online, preparing dietary plans and fitness exercises. These structures will be important in supporting you in the course of your journey, especially when you feel like giving up.

Once the preparation process is complete, you should then follow the steps which have been outlined above. Of course, the above-mentioned steps are not the Holy Grail to weight loss. As such, feel free to make any alterations and additions based on your personal needs and expectations.

If the dietary and fitness trials that you put into place do not work, do not be afraid to admit this to yourself. Do not look at them as failures, but rather as opportunities to learn and apply the acquired knowledge in the future.

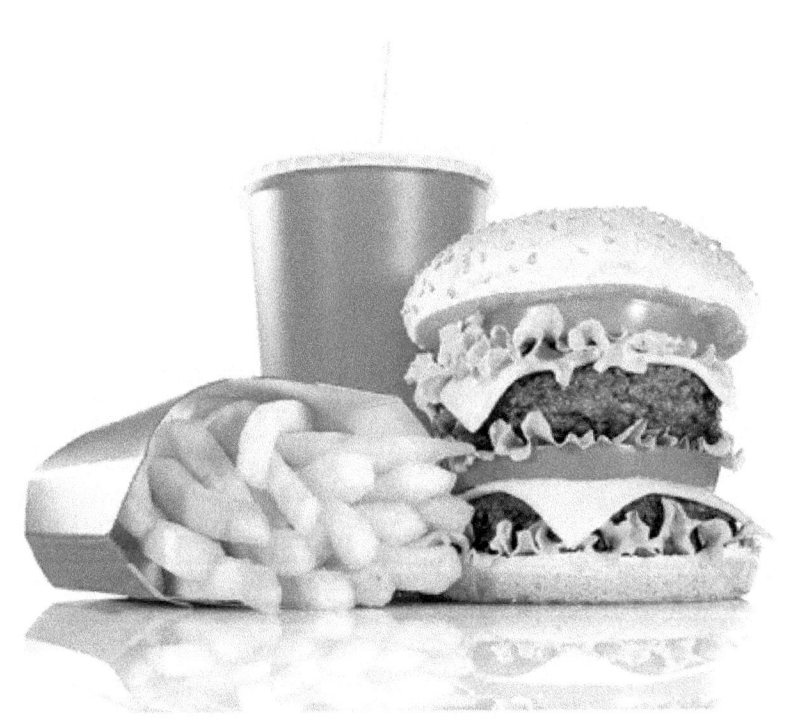

Chapter 3: The Problem with our Diet

3.1 Today's Fast Food Culture

Fast food culture began in the early 20th century with the discovery of the legendary hamburger which, at the time, was sold by the fast food chain restaurant, White Castle, and later, by the McDonald brothers. Today, there are hundreds, if not thousands of fast-food chain restaurants spread across the globe. Some of the most popular fast food restaurants include: Subway, McDonald's, Starbucks, Pizza Hut, Burger King, KFC, and Taco Bell, amongst many others.

The consumption of western-style fast food has spread widely throughout different cultures across the globe. Some of the popular fast food meals include: hamburgers, fries, fried chicken, fish, sandwiches, tacos, pizzas, hot dogs, onion rings, pitas, and ice cream. As such, the fast food industry makes billions of dollars annually and is a major employer of minimum wage workers in most developed countries.

Fast food restaurants are virtually located everywhere, from busy sidewalks and streets to airports, shopping centers, and even hospital lobbies. As such, fast foods are widely preferred due to the convenience that they offer. As opposed to spending time preparing meals, people can simply pop into the local fast food restaurant and grab a meal. Better still, one can simply order their meals from the comfort of their office or house. Due to economies of scale, fast food is considerably cheaper compared to a traditional home-cooked meal. This factor has made the fast food culture spread widely, especially amongst the poor in America.

As a result, people who are exposed to fast foods have developed an unhealthy attachment to these foods to the extent that they are unable to fathom alternative meals and dietary plans.

3.2 Why is it Important to Shift to a Healthy Diet?

If not addressed, this problem has the potential of blowing up into a global catastrophe. Today, 2 out of every 3 American adults are obese. It is forecast that in the next 10 years, 75% of all adults in the United States will be obese. To prevent this, a paradigm shift in our dietary culture is paramount.

The truth of the matter is that people are unable to control what they eat. Due to the industrial nature of food production in these restaurants, consumers are not assured of the cleanliness standards that were upheld in preparing the food. In addition, the food is usually of lower quality, mainly because it is produced in bulk in large industrial kitchens where the focus is mainly on quantity as opposed to quality.

Since the beginning of the 20th century, there has been an upward trend in the cases of obesity, both within and outside America. It is no coincidence that this trend occurred at the same time as the advent of the fast food culture. It is a widely known fact that fast food is very fattening mainly because it involves the use of very greasy and fatty ingredients.

As if this is not enough, the growth of the fast food industry has been related to lifestyle diseases such as diabetes and cardiovascular disease. According to a report by the National Research Council, more than half of known cancers have been related to high-fat diets. This implies that most, if not all, lifestyle diseases can, to a large extent, be prevented.

3.3 The Paradigm Shift from Fast Food to Healthy Food

Today, few people in developed nations regard home-made food as a proper meal. Millennials are increasingly trying out new restaurants and eating joints, as opposed to trying out traditional food recipes, which ironically are widely available. Convincing such a generation to pursue healthier food options will therefore only take place through a serious paradigm shift that will greatly affect an industry which has been in operation for more than 50 years now.

Bearing in mind the magnitude of this problem, a shift from fast food to healthy food will call for a lot of time, effort and, most of all, dedication. You will first have to realize that fast food is not merely food but a culture, a way of life that is deeply engrained in our being. Hence, you will need to take one step at a time, realizing that if you make too many changes, you will most likely get discouraged, even before you start.

It is a generally accepted principle that you will need a month to affect each dietary change. However, the process could take less than the prescribed period, or considerably more. If it does take longer, do not look down upon yourself as people are inherently different and the expected results will be worth it.

Below are some steps that you could follow to change your diet:

1. Changing Beverages

The first step in shifting from an unhealthy to a healthy diet is changing the beverages that you consume. Drinks such as sodas and sweet teas are popularly referred to as liquid calories. This is because they contain little to no nutrients and instead have high amounts of calories. Overconsumption of these drinks leads to an increase in weight.

You could begin with a goal of eliminating liquid calories within a period of one month. This will be achieved by scaling down the quantity of liquid calories that you consume. Hence, if you drink more than two bottles a day, you could begin by scaling the quantity down by several bottles. If you do not drink water, or drink very little water, you could begin by consistently increasing your water intake until you achieve the daily recommended quantity of eight glasses per day. You could boost your water intake by adding lemon slices to your mineral water to make it a little more flavorful.

2. Boost your Intake of Fruits and Vegetables

Fruits and vegetables are an important constituent of a healthy diet. They are rich in nutrients, minerals, and phytonutrients, which boost the individual's immunity and help to fight disease-causing organisms.

To transition to a healthy diet, aim to increase your daily intake of fruits and vegetables to the daily recommended quantity of 4 to 5 cups within a period of one month. This can be achieved by including fruits and vegetables in all the three meals of the day, and any snacks that you consume in the course of the day. To boost your intake, you could steam some of the vegetables or incorporate some of the fruits in your foods.

It is important to note that there are many snacks and foods whose labels begin with the word "fruit" to make consumers believe that the products are healthy. However, most of the time, the fruits are not usually the main ingredient. As such, you should avoid such products and focus on eating the actual fruit.

3. Swap the Fats you Consume

Most, if not all fast food meals contain a lot of unhealthy oils which only serve to add several pounds to your weight. Commercially manufactured snacks and baked foods contain hydrogenated oils which are meant to extend the shelf lives of these products.

Red meats are believed to contain high amounts of saturated fats. These fats are believed to lead to heart diseases, diabetes, and colorectal cancer, one of the most common types of cancer.

To transition to a healthy diet, identify and eliminate all foods that contain both hydrogenated and partially hydrogenated oils. Replace the unhealthy oils with liquid oils such as olive, coconut, and canola oils, which are healthier. You could also increase your intake of healthier fats contained in avocados, olives, cold water fish, nuts, and seeds. In food preparation, avoid frying foods and opt for the healthier methods of food preparation such as baking and broiling.

Furthermore, you should reduce your intake of red meats and instead consume white meats such as chicken, fish, and turkey which contain less saturated fats and are therefore healthier.

4. Avoid Highly Refined Foods

The standard fast food meal, and by extension, the modern-day diet, is highly grained based. It contains foods such as rice, pasta, cereals, bread, biscuits, and crackers. These foods are highly refined and stripped of their most important nutrients and fibers. The nutrients are then replaced with synthetic vitamins and high fructose corn syrup. These carbohydrates are easily converted into glucose. Hence, over-eating these foods could easily result in increased weight and type 2 diabetes.

Transitioning to a healthier diet will involve foregoing some of these carbohydrates and opting for the healthier whole grain varieties. This implies that brown bread will replace white bread, and oatmeal will replace the sugary cereals that we have for breakfast.

Your Quick Start Action Step:

In addition to following the above-mentioned steps, maintaining a food diary is also very important in your journey to healthy eating. A food diary is a powerful tool that is used to track the food that you consume in order to understand your eating habits. This information is essential when making any dietary changes and in maintaining a healthy body weight. After all, knowledge is power!

To get the most out of your food diary, you need to be as truthful as possible. Cheating to look good will do you no good. Below are some of the things that you will need to keep a record of:

- The type of food, snack, or drink:

You should note down every meal that you consume, specifying whether there were any extras such as sauces, toppings, or condiments. This will be important in identifying the trends in your eating habits, if any.

- The quantity of foods and drinks:

Write down the amounts of food or drink that you consume. You could use different methods of measuring quantities including, but not limited to: volume, weight in grams or kilograms, and counting the number of items.

- The time and venue:

Make sure to note down the time in which you consume each meal as well as the place where you eat from, either the name of the restaurant or the specific room where you eat from.

- The person that you eat with:

You should specify whether you had any company as you were eating by listing down the names of the people you were eating with, if any.

- Activities engaged in:

List any activities that you took part in as you were eating. This could include watching the television, listening to the radio, playing games, working, or even holding a conversation.

- Your mood:

Most importantly, you must specify any emotions that you experienced as you were eating. This is important as it could help you to establish a relationship, if any, between your moods and your eating habits.

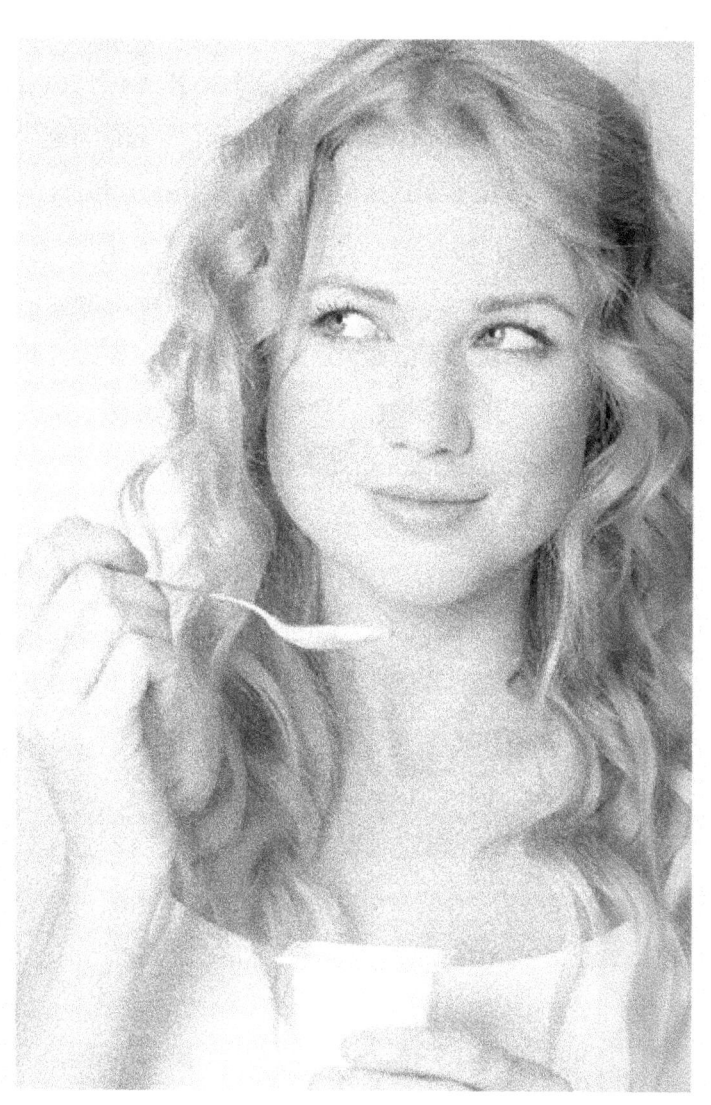

Chapter 4: Intermittent Fasting: An Overview on How to Lose Weight Faster

4.1 Expectations about the Intermittent Fasting Process

As mentioned earlier, the problem of obesity and being overweight is an issue that should be given priority in all nations across the world, with emphasis on developed nations that have adopted the western culture. Based on all the attention that this issue has been receiving, you could easily find yourself confused by the endless weight-loss strategies and dietary plans that are available in the market.

Each dietary plan and weight loss strategy is known to have its own benefits, and of course, challenges. However, none has proven to ensure efficient weight loss, while improving your longevity, as much as intermittent fasting has. As a result, the dietary plan has become very popular.

It is common practice that before you begin this dietary plan, you should visit a medical practitioner who will offer guidance on the best way to go about it. Generally, the diet is not recommended for pregnant women, women who are breastfeeding, or people with diabetes.

For those who are only beginning, the dietary plan can seem overwhelming and even impossible to some extent. There are numerous questions that you will want to ask, some of which do not have a straight answer, and which vary from one person to the next. However, we will try to shed some light on some of your burning questions.

The truth is that if you have been struggling with obesity or excessive weight, fasting can go a long way in helping you. However, you will need to keep in mind that intermittent fasting is not merely a dietary plan but a way of life. You will need to carefully plan your meals in advance depending on the method that you choose. Worse still is if you have a family, in which case you may need to have two separate meal plans.

To ensure the success of the diet, you will need to approach the whole process with a holistic view, realizing that eating a healthy diet and exercising are important pieces of the whole puzzle. You will have to avoid all junk foods and all foods rich in fats and calories or else you may find yourself gaining weight instead of losing it.

In addition, to keep track of your progress you will need tools to measure or weigh yourself. These will include: a measuring scale, a tape measure, and possibly a weight tracking application. If you do not have access to any of these, you could monitor your visual progress by frequently taking photos of your body. You could also create a spreadsheet to keep track of your diet and the changes in your body over time.

Beginners should realize they may need a little help and motivation, especially on fast days. This implies that you may need to have a bottle of water on hand. If you have difficulties getting through your first few fast days, you could indulge in less than 500 calories. If you do consume more than 500 calories, then you will need to count this as an eating day. However, do not be discouraged, the process does get easier with time.

4.2 Benefits of the Overview on the Expectations of the Intermittent Fasting Process

The above overview is very important as it will guide you through the first few days or weeks of your dietary plan. It is also meant to save you the trouble of researching every single element of the intermittent fasting dietary plan by providing you with a conclusive starter pack and a companion that will walk you through the entire journey.

According to a study that was conducted and published in the Harvard School of Public Health, the drop-out rates of the subjects who were on the intermittent fasting diet were not significantly different from those subjects on calorie restricting diets. The range of drop-outs was between 0% and 65%, implying that intermittent fasting is not necessarily easier compared to other weight loss strategies and diets.

Bearing this in mind, it becomes important to seek the guidance of a specialist as the process may get extreme in some cases. In addition, despite the challenge that the diet possesses, be encouraged every step of the journey. Rest assured that with proper discipline, you will be able to achieve your weight loss goals.

4.3 Steps to Start the Intermittent Fasting Process

Daunting as the task may seem, you must always keep in mind that the journey of a thousand miles starts with a single step. Many are the times that people will experience food cravings and hunger pangs as soon as they get on the diet. However, do bear in mind that it gets easier!

Below are some of the steps that you will need to follow when starting and following the intermittent fasting diet:

1. Consult your medical practitioner before you start. This is especially the case if you suffer from any known medical conditions, if you are pregnant, or if you are breastfeeding.
2. Decide on the intermittent fasting method that you would like to follow. As mentioned above, there are more than 7 types of intermittent fast. You must select the one that will work best for you and stick to it.
3. Keep it simple and easy. There are two possible ways that you could look at an intermittent fasting diet: a difficult and daunting duty that you owe to yourself, or simply as a self-experiment. In addition, you must break down the entire process into small and doable steps that will keep you motivated and on-track.
4. Identify the days of the week and schedule specific periods in the course of the day in which you will have your meals or fast. This will help to guide you through the process. However, the timings can always be changed depending on your schedule and bodily needs. In addition, identify a meal plan that works. Ideally, the meal plan should be high in proteins, healthy fats, fruits, and vegetables. Carbohydrates should be consumed in moderation.

5. Zero in on the primary reason that you are fasting and work towards achieving the goal. Intermittent fasting does have a myriad of benefits for your body and you do need to zero in on one specific benefit for the best results.
6. During the intermittent fasting diet, make sure to drink the recommended eight glasses of water daily. In addition, avoid foods that are rich in fats, sugars, and refined carbohydrates even during your non-fasting days. This will consistently keep your body in the fat burning state.
7. Make sure to fit fasting into your life and not the other way around. The truth is that there will be moments where it will be impossible to fast during holidays, vacations, and other forms of celebration. Nonetheless, do not limit your social interactions because of your fasting needs. Instead, take time off to celebrate with the greater community, and maybe later find a way to compensate.
8. Keep yourself busy. The one sure way to be positive that you do not feel the hunger is to keep yourself occupied. Often, you will be too busy to remember the hunger, as is the case during busy work days.
9. Ride the waves of hunger. It is scientifically proven that hunger pangs come in waves. In such moments, take a break and drink a cup of water, or a warm cup of coffee. This is because coffee is proven to be a mild appetite suppressant which will help you control your appetite.
10. Avoid snacking too much. Tempting as it may be to grab a snack during your feeding window, you must always bear in mind that small calories eventually add up. To solve this problem, make sure you set a strict calorie goal for yourself each day, and correctly count your calories to make sure that you remain within this limit.
11. During eating days or periods, avoid binge eating or feasting. It is advised that you should pretend like nothing has happened and eat based on your dietary requirements. As mentioned, the meal should be nutritious and balanced.

12. Give yourself time to fully adapt to the intermittent fasting dietary plan. This could be anywhere between a week to a month. The duration greatly varies from one person to the next. However, if you take longer, take heart, do not be discouraged, we are all different. The most important thing is that you hit your goal.
13. Gradually increase your fasting with time. Once you are on the intermittent fasting diet, you could adjust your fasting based on your body and its response to intermittent fasting. Over time, you could increase your fasting window from 14 hours to 16, or 20 hours.
14. Repeat the process. As mentioned, intermittent fasting is a way of life and you cannot expect the results to be visible within one day, one week, or even one month. The intended results will come with consistency in the pursuit of your goal.
15. Address any worries that you may have. The truth of the matter is that there are many questions that will come up in the course of the diet, some of which have answers, and some which do not. These questions have the potential of turning into worries which will make you nervous and unable to fully focus on your goal. Ergo, you should address any worries as soon as they come up. Always bear in mind that the intermittent fasting diet is not hazardous.

Your Quick Start Action Step:

To begin intermittent fasting, you must make sure that your mindset is right. Ensure that you are aware of the goal that you intend to achieve, the intermittent fasting method that you will use, and you are free of any anxiety or worries.

In addition, make sure to set aside at least 30 minutes each day to review your meal plan, clearly specifying the types of foods and drinks that you will have, if any, and the timing of your meals.

You must then follow each of the steps mentioned above and, where you have any questions, make sure to consult the advice of your doctor.

Prepare a spreadsheet and record all changes frequently to keep track of your progress. If you feel sick or nauseated, stop the intermittent fasting diet immediately and ask for medical advice before continuing.

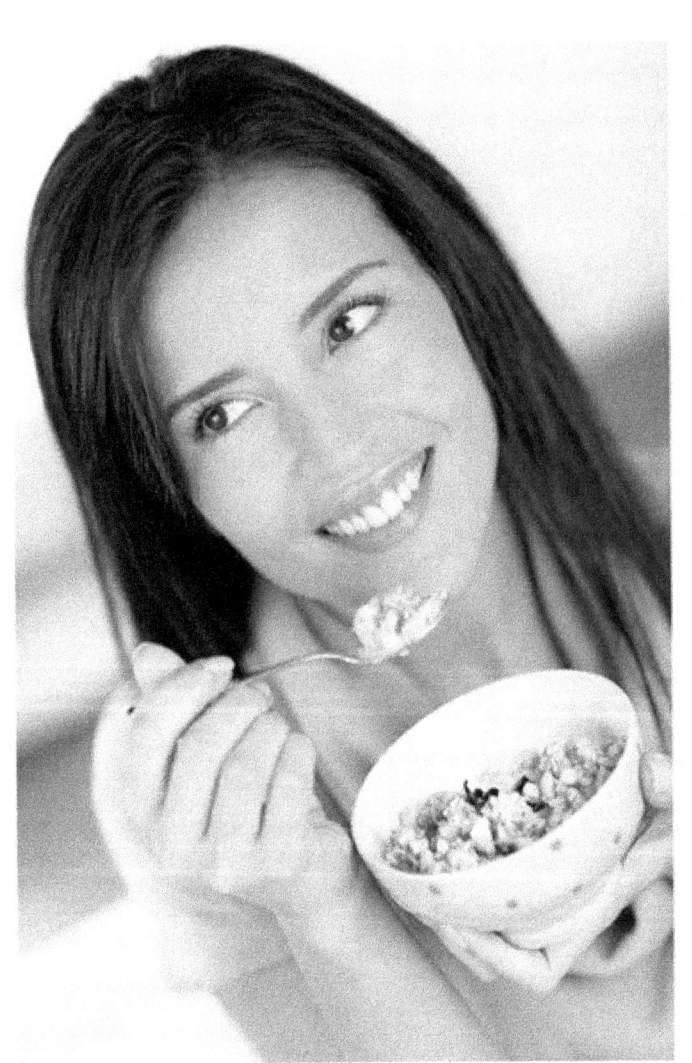

Chapter 5: Intermittent Fasting: Best Foods to Eat

5.1 What Type of Foods should be Considered for Intermittent Fasting?

Intermittent fasting, like many other dietary plans, involves the consumption of healthy and nutritious foods. The diet lays attention on both the quality and quantity of the foods that you consume to ensure that you achieve your desired goals.

Foods that are considered for intermittent fasting should contain all the important macro and micronutrients to contribute to good health and the general well-being of the person.

Foods that are high in fiber are highly recommended for intermittent fasting diets. Fiber contained in foods is broadly classified as either soluble or insoluble fiber. However, both serve the functions of: contributing to satiety, regulating the speed of digestion, and by extension, the rate at which glucose is absorbed into the bloodstream, reducing constipation and the risk of colon cancer. Fiber rich vegetables include: broccoli, cucumbers, carrots, Brussel sprouts, beetroots, spinach, kale, and celery roots, amongst others.

Foods that are rich in proteins are also highly recommended. High protein diets are important as they reduce your appetite, cravings and hunger levels, boost your metabolism and fat burning, contribute to increased muscles, and are generally good for your bones. The proteins that you consume should be low carb, and in the case of meats, lean. This is because fatty cuts of beef or pork usually contain saturated fats, which are essentially unhealthy, and could lead to increased cholesterol levels.

Fruits and vegetables are also of particular importance. Vegetables are known to contain fibers which take a long time to be digested in the gut. As such, these vegetables create a feeling of satiation, keeping hunger pangs and cravings at bay. Fruits on the other hand are rich in minerals and vitamins, which boost your general body immunity and contribute to your wellbeing.

People are advised to avoid foods that are rich in saturated fats, refined sugars, and simple carbohydrates. These include: red meats, white foods, and all foods that are prepared through deep-frying.

5.2 Why are these Foods Important in Achieving your Intermittent Fasting Goals

Eating foods that are rich in both macro and micronutrients are very important in maintaining the health and general wellbeing of the human body. In addition, while starvation is essentially the deprivation of food and important nutrients, intermittent fasting is simply a cycle of feeding and fasting. As such, the foods consumed during the feeding window should be highly nutritious or else the intermittent fasting diet will not work.

Nutrients are also important in ensuring that the biological process of autophagy is operational. Autophagy refers to the process by which the cells in the body can remove any junk in the bloodstream and recycle wastes. Malnourishment causes the autophagy process to slow down and may cause the cells to cannibalize and result in fast aging,

Foods that are rich in fiber have numerous benefits for people who are fasting intermittently. First, foods that are rich in fiber are important in preventing constipation. This is because soluble fibers absorb a lot of water, making your stool softer and larger, while insoluble fibers make your stool bulkier. As such, the stool is easily able to pass through your gut, preventing the constipated feeling.

Second, foods that are rich in fiber absorb a lot of water in the gut. They are then converted into a gel which makes the process of digestion take a longer time. This in turn has the effect of making you feel satiated for longer periods of time. Satiation then reduces the occurrence of any hunger pangs and cravings, making it easier to fast for longer periods of time.

Foods that are rich in protein are also important in contributing towards building muscle and lean tissue. Proteins contain amino acids which are important building blocks for the body. This implies that the muscles and the cells in the body require proteins to remain healthy. Hence, proteins allow you to lose weight while still maintaining some body mass. Proteins also create a feeling of satiation which allows you to go for extended periods of time without breaking your fast.

Eating a diet that is rich in vegetables is also very important since vegetables are low in fat and calories, reducing the occurrence of heart diseases. They are also important sources of nutrients which contribute to your general health. Vegetables also contain fibers, which as we have mentioned, creates a feeling of satiation and reduces constipation.

5.3 Best Foods to Try for Intermittent Fasting

1. Vegetables are some of the important foods that you will need during your intermittent fast. This is because they contain plenty of nutrients, including but not limited to: vitamin C, vitamin A, vitamin D, sodium, magnesium, potassium, and folic acid. Potassium may lower your blood pressure, decrease the chances of developing kidney stones, and reduce your bone loss. Most importantly, vegetables are low in fats and calories, which is important in your weight loss journey. Some of the common vegetables that you could add to your diet include: carrots, cabbage, cauliflower, broccoli, beetroot, spinach, kale, bell peppers, and lettuce, amongst others.
2. Like vegetables, fruits also have a myriad of benefits for your health. They contain nutrients such as: calcium, fiber, iron, magnesium, potassium, sodium, vitamin A, vitamin C, iron, and folate, amongst others. These nutrients are very important in building up the body's immunity for protection against disease-causing germs and bacteria. In addition, they are also low in fats and calories. Some of these fruits include: oranges, tangerines, lime, apples, bananas, pineapples,

mangoes, blueberries, strawberries, peaches, and grapes, amongst others. A recent study has revealed that berries are rich in flavonoids, which result in smaller increases in BMI over a 14-year period.

3. Foods that are rich in proteins are also known as body-building foods mainly because they contain important amino acids which form the building blocks of our muscles and cellular structure. Some common foods that are rich in protein and suitable for the intermittent fasting diet include: chicken breast, eggs, tofu, mushroom, lean cuts of beef, pork and lamb, legumes such as beans, peas, chickpeas, and lentils.

4. Nuts and seeds provide numerous fats, fibers, vitamins, and minerals. Some of the nutrients include: vitamin E, calcium, zinc, potassium, magnesium, manganese, and copper, amongst others. Nuts contain lots of healthy fats which create a feeling of satiation, which helps to reduce appetite and hunger. Furthermore, studies seem to suggest that consuming about 30 grams of nuts daily may reduce the risk of developing heart diseases, as well as your cholesterol levels. The fibers in nuts and seeds also reduce the reabsorption of cholesterol into the gut. Some of the recommended nuts and seeds include: almonds, walnuts, pistachios, macadamia, pumpkin seeds, sunflower seeds, and watermelon seeds.

5. Whole foods are also highly recommended for the intermittent fasting diet, and more generally as part of a healthy diet. This is because they are rich in dietary fibers and B vitamins. Dietary fibers are important for healthy bowel movements, and to reduce constipation. B vitamins are also important to release fats, proteins, and carbohydrates. Generally, whole foods are important in reducing cholesterol levels and the risk of heart diseases. Some of the whole foods that are recommended for the intermittent fasting diet include: oats, quinoa, sorghum, barley, and white rice.

6. Unsaturated fats and oils are also highly recommended for the intermittent fasting diet. The fats and oils are healthy and contribute to the feeling of satiation, which is important if you are going to be

fasting for extended periods of time. Some of the common sources of healthy fats and oils include: olive oil, coconut oil, peanut butter, almond butter, and sunflower butter, amongst others.

Your Quick Start Action Step:

Before starting the intermittent fasting diet, you should check your pantry and refrigerator to make sure that you have some of these foods and the ingredients that will be required to make a meal that is in line with the intermittent fasting diet. If you do not have some of these foods, make sure to visit your local grocery store to stock your pantry.

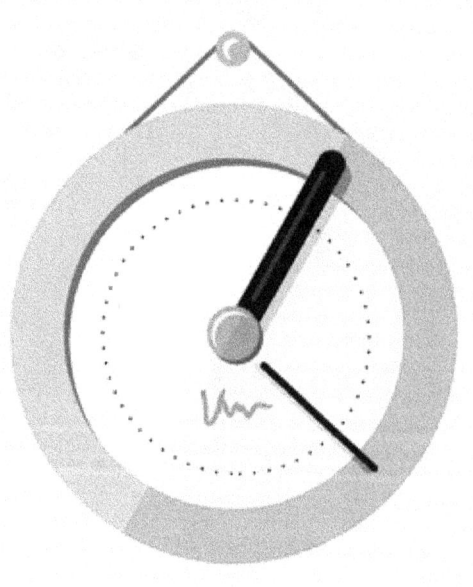

Chapter 6: Intermittent Fasting: Best Time to Eat in a Day

6.1 The Relevance of the Time of Day when Intermittent Fasting
It is a widely shared opinion that it does not matter what time of day you decide to eat. What matters most in determining whether you gain or lose weight is the type, amount of food, and the amount of physical activity that you engage in during the day. As accurate as this may sound, it is sadly a myth, one that has become widely popularized over time.

The truth of the matter is that the time of day is extremely important in determining the success of your intermittent fast. Many folks will advise you against eating large meals in the evening, stating that you will not get the opportunity to burn off the food, causing it to be stored in the body as fat. While this may not be true in the strict sense, there is evidence that links obesity to feeding on heavy meals at night.

The best time to have your eating window, and by extension, the largest meal of the day, is any time between noon and 3:00 pm. People who finish their calories for the day by 3:00 pm have improved insulin sensitivity, lower blood pressure, and reduced hunger pangs and cravings.

This approach is effective because the body follows a natural circadian rhythm in which it burns fuel during the day, then enters storage mode during the night. As such, when people finish their calories by 3:00 pm, they will have burnt glucose and fat during the day and there will be no fats to be stored in the body at night.

In addition, the natural circadian rhythm of the ghrelin hormone leads to increased hunger at night. Having your last meal by 3:00 pm therefore becomes beneficial, as it prevents people from consuming excessive calories, especially at night, when people find it most difficult to control their food intake due to increased hunger.

Limiting our feeding to these hours is extremely beneficial as we can control our blood pressure and blood sugar. Our hormonal control becomes better leading to improved disease prevention and reduced inflammation in the body. In addition, you will sleep better as you will go to bed with little hunger. This will reduce the occurrence of stomach upsets, heartburns, and feelings of being too full, which are associated with poor sleeping patterns.

6.2 The Rationale Behind Time of Day
- The human body, like the bodies of other animals, has been scientifically proven to operate in circadian rhythms. These are cyclical changes in behavior and hormones which occur every 24 hours.
- The circadian rhythms govern all hormones, including but not limited to: growth hormones, parathyroid hormones, insulin, and ghrelin. Of importance in this case is insulin, which is proven to contribute to weight gain, and ghrelin, which is a hormone that controls hunger.
- Ghrelin rises and falls based on the natural circadian rhythm. Hunger, which is controlled by the ghrelin hormone, also rises and falls based on the natural circadian rhythm. The ghrelin hormone is usually lowest early in the morning, at about 8:00 am and highest later in the evening at about 8:00 pm.
- Correspondingly, hunger is lowest early in the morning at about 7:50 am and highest in the evening at around 7:50 pm. Hence, we see that hormones are key in the regulation of hunger.
- At 7:50 am, hunger is low. It therefore makes no sense to force ourselves to feed. At 7:50 pm, hunger is maximally stimulated, implying that the more food you consume, the higher the insulin levels in your bloodstream, and the greater the weight gain.

- Since the hormonal regulation of hunger is independent of the fast/eat cycle in an intermittent fasting diet, it becomes important to establish an optimal strategy that will determine the best time to have the largest meal of the day.
- Bearing this in mind, the optimal strategy becomes eating the largest meal between noon and 3:00 pm. Hence, implying that individuals on an intermittent fasting diet should schedule their eating windows during this time.

6.3 Steps to Follow

It is true that the concept of a limited feeding period with prolonged periods of fasting may terrify you greatly. To you, the concept of fasting may be synonymous to starvation and may invoke feelings of suffering and anguish. Worse still, you probably cannot fathom why you should avoid eating food. Yet it is right there, tempting you to eat it. The idea of going a whole day without food may even be incomprehensible to you.

However, I assure you that the intermittent fasting diet is indeed doable. This method, for lack of a better word, could be referred to as the 21/3 method. In this method, you get to fast for a period of 24 hours and only get to eat food in a 3-hour window between noon and 3:00 pm. The method could also be applied during alternate-day fasting.

Below are the steps to follow when implementing an intermittent fasting diet where the feeding window is optimally scheduled between noon and 3:00 pm:

1. On the day that you choose to begin your intermittent fasting diet, enjoy your last meal of the day between noon and 3:00 pm. After this meal, you will begin calculating your fasting hours beginning from 3:00 pm.
2. Proceed with your day, only drinking water, unsweetened tea, and coffee whenever you experience a pang of hunger. When the night falls and evening comes, make sure to sleep for 8 hours. By the time

you wake up, you will have completed more than half of your fasting period.

3. If you really cannot make it until morning, it is highly recommended that you consume a light meal that is high in protein, such as a protein shake or a few carbs. This meal is best eaten at least one hour before you go to bed. It is important as it will supply you with all the important nutrients while keeping your stomach full and free of hunger or cravings.

4. Based on the natural circadian rhythm of the human body, you are less likely to feel hungry in the morning. In addition, if you had a proper meal the previous day, the chances of feeling hungry are even lower. However, you can always drink some mineral water, unsweetened tea, or coffee if you do experience any hunger. If you really cannot make it to noon, you can have a smoothie or a light meal to break your fast. However, if you can take it, push yourself to noon without eating any solid food.

Your Quick Start Action Step:

Having gone through the above steps, I believe that you are confident that you can implement the intermittent fasting diet above. You will need to have prepared a dietary plan in advance, which you will use to dictate the meals that you have during these periods. The meals will need to be rich in proteins, fruits and vegetables, and low in carbohydrates, as per the intermittent fasting diet.

The final and most important thing will then be to schedule a time between noon and 3:00 pm to have your meals. While having your meals, avoid eating in a hurry, as you will be more likely to over-eat. Eating slowly creates a feeling of fullness in your stomach, which limits the amount of food that you consume.

However, to ensure the success of this intermittent fasting diet, you must let go of the notion that has long been embedded in us that dinner is the most important meal of the day. You will need to reprogram your thinking, which, though difficult, is very possible. With reduced pressure to prepare a large meal for dinner, you will have more time to yourself to spend on other activities that equally need your attention.

While our social needs and demands may make it difficult to have the last meal of the day before 3:00 pm, you must always believe that where there is a will, there is a way. In addition, you must remember that the intermittent fasting diet is meant to fit into your life and not the other way around. Hence, do not restrict your social interactions based on this diet. First enjoy yourself, then later strategize on how to compensate.

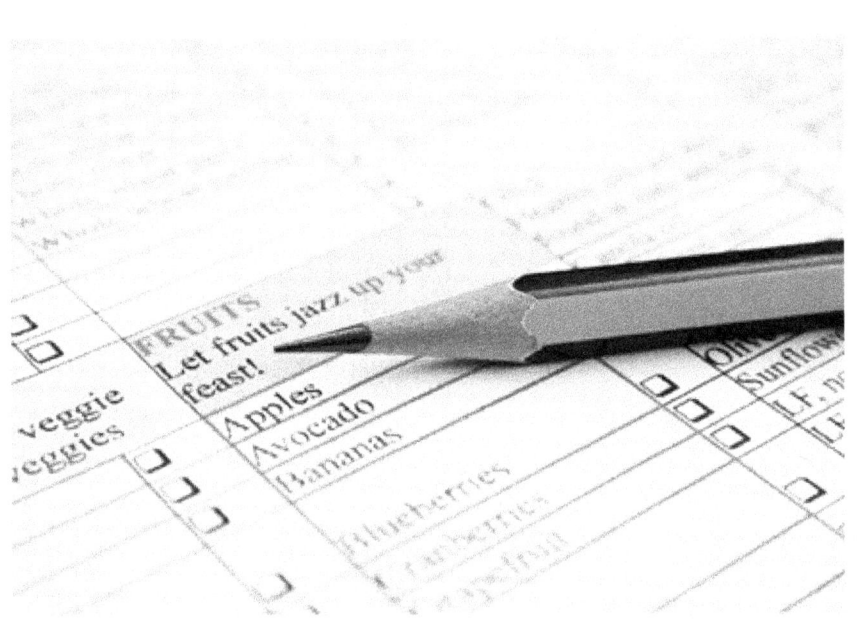

Chapter 7: Picking the Right Meal Plan

7.1 Picking the Right Meal Plan

Now that you have heard all about the intermittent fasting diet, all that remains is learning about how you can prepare a seven-day meal plan. Depending on the method of intermittent fasting that you follow, there are different foods and drinks that you could combine to form a unique meal plan that will suit your dietary needs. In this case, we will focus on the 16/8 method that involves restricting the hours in which you can eat.

It is medically recommended that the meal plan should contain several small meals and snacks which are evenly spread out within the eating window. The meal plan should not allow for binge eating or feasting but should control the portions of food and snacks that one eats at each point in time, depending on the level of hunger.

To maximize the potential health benefits and to ensure weight loss, it is important to stick to a nutritious diet. You should avoid all manner of junk foods, foods that are rich in sugar and simple carbohydrates, and all white and refined foods.

Ideally, the best meal plan should contain: foods that are rich in soluble fibers such as nuts, beans, fruits, and vegetables. Foods that are rich in protein such as meat, fish, nuts and tofu, whole grains such as oats, barley, quinoa, and buckwheat, vegetables such as broccoli, cauliflower, cucumbers, and tomatoes. Also, foods that are rich in healthy fats and oils such as nuts, seeds, and even fish.

The meal plan should also include beverages that are free of calories, such as mineral water, unsweetened teas and coffees, or cinnamon teas.

7.2 The Importance of Picking the Right Meal Plan

The right meal plan should consist of small meals and snacks that are spread out during the eating period. This is important in keeping hunger under control by preventing excessive hunger pangs. The prevention of excessive hunger pangs also reduces the likelihood of binge eating and feasting.

In addition, due to the small, but high, frequency of the meals, the blood sugar levels are maintained at a relatively constant level, preventing the occurrence of insulin resistance or high blood pressure.

The right meal plan should be nutritious for the success of the intermittent fasting diet. Nutritious meals contain all the important proteins, carbohydrates, vitamins, and minerals for the healthy development of the person. Any meal plan that is not nutritious is more likely to lead to weight gain than it is likely to lead to weight loss.

The presence of soluble fibers in a meal plan is important, especially during intermittent fasting as it creates a feeling of being full, preventing any hunger pangs that may occur. During digestion, the soluble fibers attract a lot of water, turning into gel and slowing down the digestion process, hence creating the feeling of being full.

Foods that are rich in protein are also important, as they provide the body's muscles with all the protein nutrients that are required for healthy growth, while keeping the stomach full and preventing hunger pangs.

The right meal plan should also contain whole foods, as opposed to white foods. This is because white foods are highly refined and contain synthetic vitamins, while whole foods are not refined, contain no synthetic vitamins, and are therefore highly nutritious.

Calorie-free drinks such as water are important as they are not only used to remain hydrated, but also to control hunger and appetite for food. Black unsweetened coffee is particularly important, as it boosts the metabolism of the body, increasing the rate at which glucose and fats are turned into energy.

Raw fruits and vegetables are particularly important, as they contain the soluble fibers which create a feeling of being full. In addition, they contain important vitamins and minerals, which are utilized by the body to boost its immunity.

7.3 Steps on Picking the Right Meal Plan

While using the 16/8 method of intermittent fasting, you will need to schedule an eight-hour eating period at a time of your own choosing. However, you should keep in mind that the optimal time to eat is usually between noon and 3:00 pm in line with the natural circadian rhythm.

Below are some of the steps that you will need to follow to identify the right meal plan:

1. Ideally, you should begin your day without any carbohydrates in your system. This is done to ensure that the body is in a state of ketosis where it is burning fats to produce energy rather than glucose.

2. The meals of the day should be spread out across the 8-hour period depending on the dietary needs, hunger, and the activities that you will engage in at a particular point in time. For example, you could divide the feeding window into 3 distinct meal plans which are equally spaced out.

3. In addition, you could consume coffee every morning to boost your metabolism, reduce your appetite, and give you a positive mood and stamina. The daily recommended amount of coffee that you can consume within a day is 2 – 3 small cups. You could drink coffee during your fasting window to reduce any hunger pangs that you may experience.

4. You should have the first meal of the day within 3 – 4 hours after waking up. Pushing this meal later into the day forces the body to burn up some of its fat reserves to generate energy without relying on glucose from food. You should have the last meal of the day 3 – 4 hours before you retire to bed. Based on the natural circadian rhythm of the ghrelin hormone, this ensures that you do not eat food at a point in which the body is storing up its reserves as it might lead to weight gain.

5. The first meal of the day, which is meant to break the fast, is supposed to be very healthy and modest in size. Breaking the fast with a very large meal or through binge eating will slow down the fat burning process in your body, making you tired in the late hours of the morning. The first meal should contain 300 – 400 calories and should generally contain some protein, healthy fats, and fruits. Some of the foods that you could eat at this point include: canned tuna, an omelet, chicken breast, berries, apples, avocados, almond milk, protein shakes, and some almond nuts.

6. Your second and third meals of the day should each contain about 500 – 600 calories and should be high in protein and with moderate amounts of fats and carbohydrates. An example of such a meal would be: chicken breast, some yam wedges, veggies, and blueberries.

7. You should always keep in mind that intermittent fasting is a dietary plan that restricts your eating to certain periods in the course of the day or the week. Hence, if you successfully complete your fasting period but consume twice, or thrice, the amount of food and calories that you are supposed to, your fast will essentially be pointless and could result in weight gain and feelings of fatigue. Hence, both food quality, and food quantity, must be honored.

8. All meals that you consume should contain healthy portions of both soluble and insoluble fibers. This is because fibers quickly absorb water once they enter the digestive system. They then turn into gel, which is digested slowly, creating a feeling of fullness. In addition, fiber does reduce constipation. Fiber is mainly contained in foods such as broccoli, cauliflower, and Brussels sprouts.

9. Berries are also an important addition to your meal plan. They are believed to contain healthy portions of vital vitamins and nutrients, which boost your immunity and contribute to your general wellbeing. It is scientifically proven that people who consume

healthy portions of strawberries and blueberries experience smaller increases in BMI over a 14-year period.
10. Any snacks that you consume should not contain carbohydrates. They should mainly include coffee, green tea, apples, or even some nuts.
11. Fish is highly recommended as it contains healthy fats, proteins, and vitamin D. Because of this, fish has long been considered a 'brain food', as it highly nourishes the body and, by extension, the brain.
12. Probiotics are also important constituents of your meal plan. The enzymes and bacteria in the body thrive on consistency and diversity. Hence, when you feel hungry, you may experience some side effects, such as constipation. Probiotic rich foods and supplements are therefore important in ensuring that the enzymes and bacteria responsible for digestion are satisfied, preventing any side effects.
13. Once you have identified your fasting and feeding windows, you should try to keep these periods constant, since hunger is controlled by the ghrelin hormone, which follows the circadian cycle. Hence, after some weeks, you will realize that you will experience hunger at specific points in time, and it is best to maintain this regular pattern.
14. Leguminous plants are also very important in your intermittent fasting diet. Legumes such as beans, peas, chickpeas, lentils, and even black beans, are low-calorie carbohydrates which are very important in your intermittent fasting diet.
15. While preparing a meal plan, some of the foods that you should avoid at all costs include: refined starches, white foods, added sugars, trans fats, and processed foods.

Your Quick Start Action Step:

Coming up with a meal plan that is suited to the intermittent fasting diet is a process that will require you to schedule significant amounts of time to conduct in depth research, to consult with your doctor, and to source for all the materials that you need.

You should keep in mind that the foods that you include in your meal plan should be low-calorie and nutrient-dense foods that will nourish your muscles and organs, while allowing your body to burn down fats to release energy. It may be difficult to list down all the foods that you can eat, however, as a general guideline, you should focus on: lean proteins, plant proteins, fruits, vegetables, nuts, and seeds.

The key to losing weight, therefore, involves a healthy and well-balanced diet that ensures constant energy levels for the body to carry out its normal functions. Most importantly, consistency and sticking to the diet is important for the intermittent fasting diet to be successful.

As a disclaimer, if your meal plan makes you dizzy or weak, you are advised to terminate the meal plan immediately, and to seek the guidance of a nutritionist or a medical practitioner.

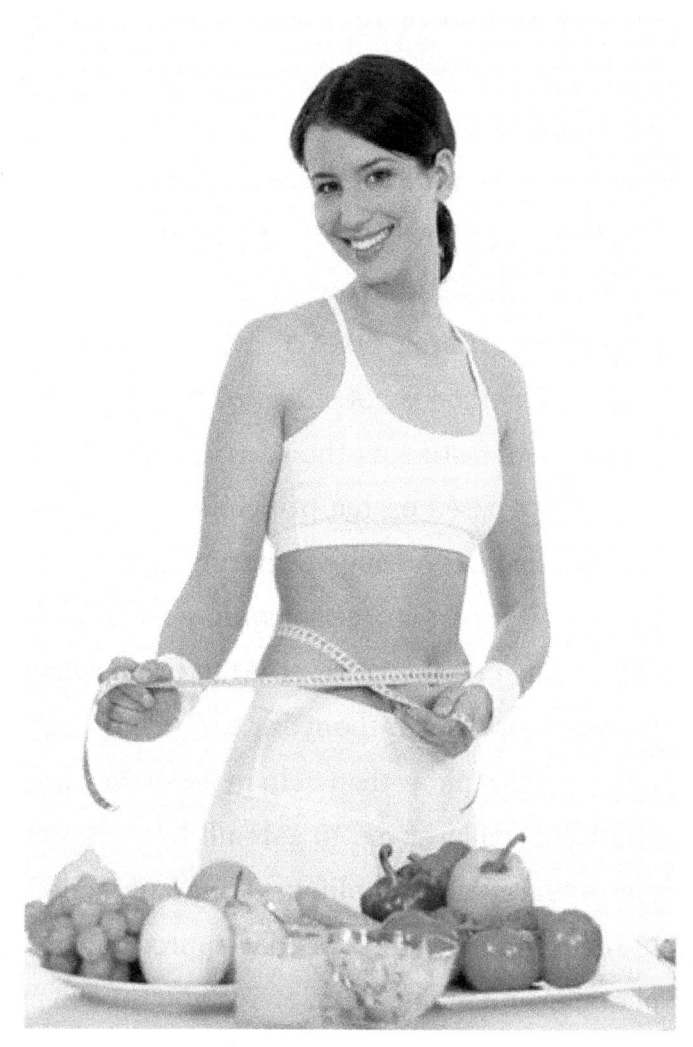

Chapter 8: The One Meal a Day Approach

8.1 Background Information

Today, intermittent fasting is one of the most powerful tools that you could use to optimize your anatomy and biology, while still shedding off some extra pounds. The methods of intermittent fasting range from calorie restriction in the course of the day, to alternating between regular feeding days and fasting days, to limiting the number of hours that you get to eat within the day.

The One Meal a Day Approach (OMAD) is a form of intermittent fasting in which you get to fast for a 23-hour window and get to eat during a one hour feeding window every single day. Unlike the other methods of intermittent fasting, OMAD shrinks the feeding window even further. As such, the method is not suitable for beginners, as it is an extreme form of intermittent fasting, or the Warrior Diet method of intermittent fasting.

The diet is based on the principles of calorie restriction and consuming low-calorie diets during one particular time of the day or night. This then allows you to fast for the remaining 23 hours of the day. The body is then able to burn up the fat reserves to produce energy, consequently leading to weight loss. Any carbohydrates or fruit sugars that are consumed during the feeding window then help in fat mobilization.

The OMAD allows you to gain all the benefits of an intermittent fasting diet, while greatly simplifying your daily schedule. This is because, unlike the conventional 3 meal per day approach, you will spend less time in meal planning and preparation, giving you time to engage in other activities.

Most dieters will have their feeding window during dinner time, since it is at this time that we experience maximum hunger, in line with the natural circadian rhythm of the ghrelin hormone. In addition, you could have unsweetened black coffee or tea in the course of the day to take care of any hunger pangs, and to suppress your appetite. You could also have an apple or an egg during the day.

8.2 Why does the OMAD Method Work?

The OMAD is considered to be an unconventional method of losing weight. The idea of having one meal per day is considered excessive and unnecessary. Hence, many people cringe at the idea of the OMAD.

However, before you make your conclusion and dismiss the diet, the proponents of OMAD highlight several benefits that are associated with this approach.

From an evolutionary standpoint, human beings engaged in food-seeking activities, which would last anywhere from a couple of hours to a few days. Human beings then developed powerful mechanisms and adaptations which allowed their bodies, and by extension, brains, to function at their optimal levels despite the scarcity in food.

The mechanisms that allowed humans to survive such periods of fasting are believed to have numerous benefits, which have been negated by the present-day sedentary lifestyle characterized by continuous and abundant food supply.

Through the OMAD, the body is supercharged by activating the stress response pathways, which boost mitochondrial performance, the body's metabolism, the production of hormones (such as growth hormones), the repair of DNA in your cells, and prevent the occurrence of chronic diseases such as: diabetes, high blood pressure, and insulin resistance. In addition, OMAD activates autophagy, the mechanism that the body uses to clean up damaged cells, toxins, and wastes.

As mentioned above, the OMAD provides for one meal each day. This implies that the intake of calories is generally very restricted compared to other individuals who eat throughout the day. Furthermore, it becomes impossible for one to have a surplus of calories, even when consuming unhealthy foods. Hence, the approach is very efficient in weight loss.

In addition, many people who follow the conventional 'three meals a day' approach can attest to the sluggish feeling that one experiences after having their lunch. As the digestion process proceeds, people experience a groggy feeling, slowing down their general productivity. Hence, the proponents of this method believe that the approach eliminates the sluggishness that people experience in the afternoon.

8.3 Steps to Follow When Doing the OMAD Approach

The OMAD approach can be very tasking, to say the least. You will need a lot of effort, discipline, and commitment if you are to succeed in this method of intermittent fasting. In addition, avoiding food for 23 hours straight will require you to reprogram your thinking away from the typical 'three meals per day' approach.

Below are some of the steps that you will need to follow to get onto the OMAD approach:

1. Consult your medical practitioner before you start. This is especially the case if you suffer from any known medical conditions, if you are pregnant, or if you are breastfeeding.
2. Identify the primary reason that you are fasting using the OMAD approach, and work towards achieving that goal. Intermittent fasting does have a myriad of benefits for your body and you do need to zero in on one specific benefit for the best results.
3. Identify and schedule the one hour that will form your feeding window. The optimal feeding window is scientifically proven to be between noon and 3:00 pm, based on the natural circadian rhythm. However, you could also schedule your one-hour feeding window in the evening, such that it coincides with dinner time, the time in which we experience the most hunger. Regardless of the window that you select, consistency is key.
4. Take one step at a time. The truth of the matter is that the OMAD approach is not as easy as the snap of a finger. You will need to slowly ease into the OMAD diet at your own pace. It is recommended that you break down the entire process into small and doable steps, which will keep you highly motivated. Since people are inherently different, it is also likely that different people

will take different durations of time to fully transition into the OMAD diet. Despite this, be encouraged to run your own race. After all, what matters is that you eventually achieve your goal.

5. Cut down on the amount of carbohydrates that you consume. When you eat lots of carbohydrates and starches, you increase the amount of glucose that is released into the bloodstream. Any excess glucose will then be converted into glycogen and stored in the liver. As such, it will take a long period of time for the body to fully shift to the fat-burning mode which is required for weight loss. In addition, a low-carb diet will keep you satisfied for longer, while reducing your appetite, and the crankiness that is associated with foods that are rich in starch.

6. Because of the extreme calorie restriction under the OMAD diet, you can virtually eat unhealthy foods, and your calorie intake will still be way below that of a person who eats three meals a day. To many people, this implies that you can eat anything you want. However, it is important to note that just because you can eat anything does not mean that you should. Your meal will still need to be well-balanced, and nutritious enough to contribute to your good health and general wellbeing.

7. Some of the meals that you should focus on eating include, but are not limited to: plant proteins, lean meats, eggs, dairy products, nuts, seeds, healthy fats and oils, whole foods, and different herbs and spices. The main foods that you should avoid include: white refined foods, cashew nuts, fatty meats, vegetable oil, butter, margarine, mayonnaise, soft drinks, and energy drinks.

8. The perfect meal plan should therefore contain, but is not limited to: at least five types of vegetables, three types of fruits, lean meats, unsalted nuts, buttermilk to aid in digestion, dark chocolate, and mineral water to remain hydrated. The meal plan should contain a wide range of both macro and micronutrients to keep your body

fully nourished. Feeding on one nutrient will therefore do you no good.

9. When you initially begin the OMAD diet, you will not have the physical or mental energy to work out because of the long fasting hours. However, you could still engage in light stretching exercises and yoga sessions to keep your muscles active. Once you get the hang of the intermittent fasting diet, you could include toning exercises to keep your skin from sagging. Alternatively, you could consult a fitness expert to structure a weight loss program for you.

10. It can be argued that the most important aspect of effecting the OMAD diet is developing the discipline and willpower to stick to the diet despite the cravings and hunger pangs that you are likely to experience. This is because hunger is a powerful feeling that can demotivate and disorient you. You will need to overcome the habit of having three meals per day by persistently convincing yourself that you can do it.

Your Quick Start Action Step:

Schedule some time to carry out in depth research and to consult a medical practitioner to provide you with all the knowledge that you will need before starting the OMAD diet. This is especially so if you are suffering from any known medical condition, if you are pregnant, or breastfeeding.

Armed with the necessary knowledge, you could follow the steps highlighted above to come up with the timing of your feeding window, a suitable meal plan, and any workouts that you plan to engage in. You will need to go out and shop for some of these foods and ingredients to restock your refrigerator and kitchen cabinets.

As you pursue this journey, you will need to realize that it will test your will and determination countless times. Hence, you will need to constantly motivate yourself and keep the company of positive people, preferably people who are pursuing the same goal. You could also frequently track your progress by recording it in a spreadsheet.

If you feel weak, dizzy, sluggish, constantly tired, or experience some brain fog, you may need to stop the OMAD diet and seek the advice of your medical practitioner. You will need to realize that all bodies are fundamentally different, and you could still achieve your intended goals with a mild form of intermittent fasting.

Nonetheless, the OMAD diet is an effective diet mainly because it helps you to prevent any future weight gain.

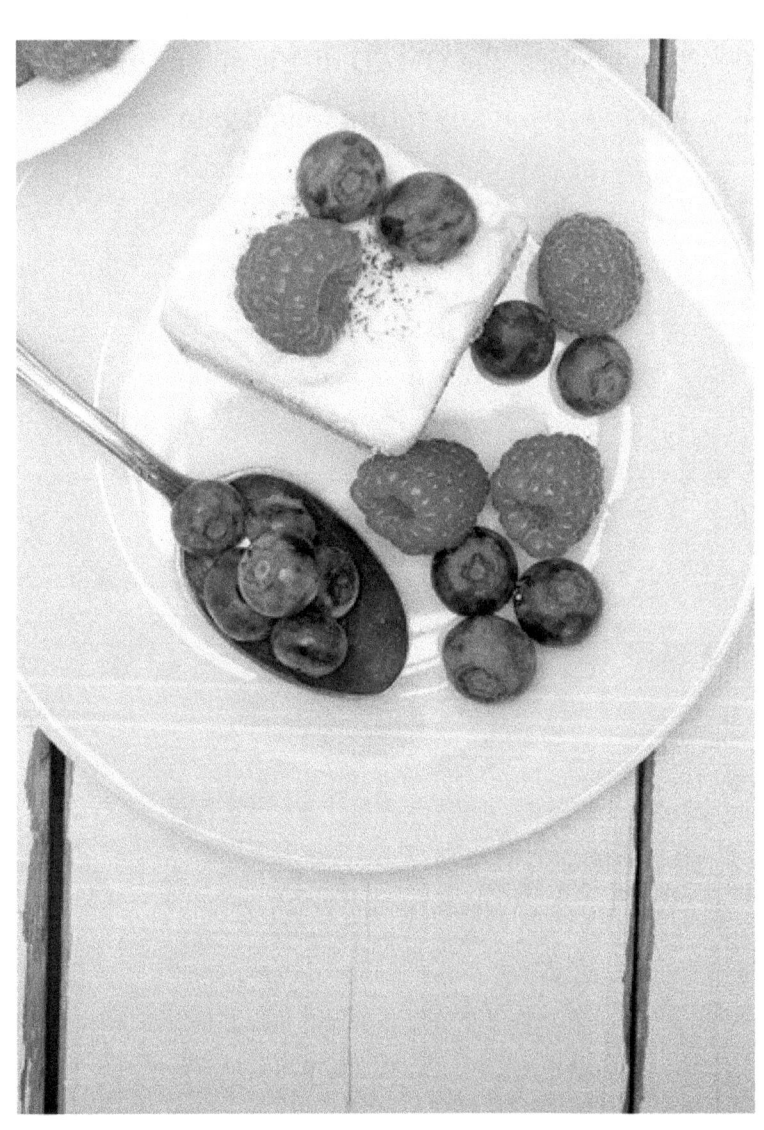

Chapter 9: Healthy Recipes

9.1 Healthy Recipes During Intermittent Fasting

Intermittent fasting has everything to do with calorie restriction just as much as it has everything to do with restricting the hours in which an individual can consume meals. As such, food quality is just as important as food quantity.

Successful weight loss using the intermittent fasting diet necessitates the use of a three-step approach that consists of a positive mindset, physical activity, exercises, and healthy and nutritious recipes.

Healthy recipes ensure that although the calorie intake is greatly restricted, the body and its vital organs by extension receives all the important macro and micronutrients.

Feeding on unhealthy meals that consist of soft drinks, energy drinks, meals that are rich in simple starches, saturated fats and oils, and white foods is extremely detrimental to your body and may cause you to gain weight as opposed to losing it.

There are many foods that you could choose from to make a delicious meal that is still in line with the intermittent fasting diet. Below are some of the foods that constitute a healthy recipe:

Vegetables such as: broccoli, cauliflower, cucumber, tomatoes, beetroot, turnips, scallions, lettuce, bell peppers, spinach, and kales. These vegetables are best eaten raw or lightly steamed or boiled to avoid destroying important nutrients and vitamins.

Fruits such as: apples, bananas, grapes, strawberries, blueberries, lemon, lime, oranges, tangerines, pineapples, peaches, plums, gooseberries, and acai berries are also very important.

Nuts and seeds such as: almonds, walnuts, pistachios, pecan, macadamia, sunflower seeds, pumpkin seeds, and melon seeds.

Proteins from foods such as: chicken breast, lean cuts of pork and beef, tofu, eggs, beans, peas, black peas, and chickpeas.

Whole grains from foods such as: brown rice, oat, millet, quinoa, barley, and sorghum. These are cereals that are hardly refined.

Dairy products such as: buttermilk, full-fat milk, full-fat yogurt, cottage cheese, cheddar cheese, and ricotta cheese.

Healthy fats and oils from foods such as: olive oil, peanut butter, coconut oil, almond butter, avocados, and sunflower butter.

Healthy calorie-free beverages such as: unsweetened teas, coffees, homemade lemonade, coconut water, freshly made fruit juices, and most importantly, mineral water.

Some of the foods that you should avoid at all costs include: fatty cuts of beef and pork, flavored yogurt, cream cheese, white grains, vegetable oil, margarine, and mayonnaise.

9.2 Why do We Need Nutritious Recipes?

Nutritious recipes are meals that contain all the important macro and micronutrients that are required by the body. Each meal should have a healthy portion of these nutritious recipes, implying that the meal should not be too big, nor too small.

Nutritious recipes are often rich in fruits and vegetables. It is highly recommended that each recipe should contain at least three different types of fruits, and three different types of vegetables. This is because fruits and vegetables are very rich in both soluble and insoluble fibers. These fibers usually take a longer time to be digested, creating a feeling of fullness and reducing hunger pangs. In addition, insoluble fibers are important in preventing constipation. Fruits often contain plenty of vitamins and minerals which are important in improving the immunity of the body. Some fruits, such as the avocado, are rich in non-saturated fats which are extremely filling and satiating.

Furthermore, nutritious recipes often contain whole grains and foods. These are important because, unlike the white grains, they are not refined. This implies that they do not contain any synthetic vitamins and minerals. The intermittent fasting diet is usually rich in proteins and fats and oils. To ensure that the diet is healthy and nutritious, nuts and seeds are used since they contain healthy fats and oils, which are important in keeping the body in a state of ketosis.

Proteins obtained from lean cuts of beef, pork, and bacon are also very important, since they contain healthy and nutritious protein, and most of the important amino acids. These proteins serve to strengthen your muscles and body organs, while keeping the glucose levels in the bloodstream low. In addition, proteins also reduce cravings and feelings of hunger, which are important in ensuring the success of an intermittent fasting diet.

Calorie-free beverages are also very important, as they provide you with the desired hydration to keep your body in perfect shape. Coffee is particularly considered to be very important, as it increases the metabolism of the body, leading to the increased burning of fat as a source of energy. In addition, coffee is important in reducing hunger pangs and cravings.

9.3 Some Healthy Recipes that you can Try During Intermittent Fasting

There are different recipes that you could try out at different times in the course of your feeding window or feeding day. These recipes will greatly depend on your dietary needs and physical activity at a particular point in time.

When breaking your fast, you should prepare meals that are rich in healthy fats but still low in calories. You should avoid binge eating or eating sugary foods when breaking your fast, as this has the potential to tire you out. Below are some of the recipes that you could try out when breaking your fast:

Recipe 1: Green Smoothie

Ingredients:

1 avocado

1 cup of coconut milk

1 handful of berries

1 cup of spinach or kale

1 cup of chia seeds

Method:

Place all the ingredients in a blender and blend until you achieve the desired consistency.

Recipe 2: Nut and Berry Parfait

Ingredients

6 crushed almonds

6 crushed walnuts

10 diced strawberries

1/3 cup blackberries

1/3 cup raspberries

½ tablespoon chia seeds

1 teaspoon cinnamon

1 teaspoon pure vanilla extract

½ cup heavy whipping cream

Method:

1. Place the whipping cream in a bowl and add the vanilla extract.
2. Use a hand mixer on medium and whip the whipped cream for about 2 to 3 minutes, or until stiff peaks form.
3. Stir the nuts and berries into the whipped cream.
4. Add in the chia seeds and sprinkle some cinnamon on the top.

Recipe 3: Grain-free Pancakes

Ingredients:

¼ cup of coconut flour

½ teaspoon of baking powder

1/4 teaspoon of salt

½ cup of whipped cream

7. eggs

1 teaspoon vanilla extract

½ tablespoon of organic honey

1 tablespoon butter

Ground cinnamon

Method:

1. Preheat the skillet over medium heat.
2. In a bowl, mix the eggs, vanilla and cream.
3. In a separate bowl, mix the coconut flour, baking soda and salt then gently stir in the wet ingredients into the dry ingredients.
4. Melt the butter in a skillet.
5. Pour about 2 to 3 tablespoons of butter into the skillet to form pancakes that are at least 10 cm in diameter.
6. Cook the pancakes for 2 -3 minutes on each side until golden brown.
7. Repeat the process until all the batter is over.

Below are some of the recipes that you could prepare for all other meals after you break your fast:

Recipe 4: Salmon and vegetables

Salmon is a type of fish that is rich in omega-3 oils, which are healthy fats that are nutritious.

Ingredients:

1 pound of salmon

2 tablespoons of lemon juice

2 tablespoons of ghee

4 cloves of garlic

Method:

1. Preheat the oven to 400°C

2. In a bowl, mix the lemon juice, ghee, and finely diced garlic.

3. Place the salmon in foil and pour the mixture above it.

4. Wrap the salmon in the foil and place it in a baking sheet.

5. Bake in the oven for 15 minutes or until the salmon is cooked. You could also roast your vegetables in a separate baking sheet or alongside the salmon.

Recipe 5: Grain-free Cauliflower Pizza

Ingredients:

1 pound of pizza florets

2 eggs, lightly beaten

1 teaspoon salt

1 teaspoon dried oregano

1 teaspoon garlic powder

Pizza toppings of your choice

Method:

1. Pre-heat the oven to 400°C.
2. Place the cauliflower in a food processor and pulse them until they are finely chopped, then transfer them to a large bowl.
3. In the bowl, add the eggs, salt, oregano and garlic powder and mix well.
4. Transfer the cauliflower mixture onto the baking sheet and spread it to form the pizza crust.
5. Bake the crust for about 20 minutes, or until the crust is slightly golden.
6. Add your desired toppings then bake for 10 – 15 minutes.

Recipe 6: Chicken Drumsticks Wrapped in Bacon

Ingredients:

4 Chicken drumsticks

4 slices of bacon

1 ½ teaspoons of salt

1 teaspoon of ground pepper

Method:

1. Pre-heat the oven to 400°F. Line the baking sheet with aluminum foil.
2. Wrap a piece of bacon around the drumstick from the bottom to the top. Place the 4 drumsticks on the baking sheet and season with salt and pepper.
3. Bake for 45 minutes or until the bacon looks golden.

Recipe 7: Strawberry and Kale Salad

Ingredients:

4 cups of kale

1 cup of walnuts

12 strawberries

1 tablespoon balsamic vinegar

4 tablespoons extra virgin oil

Salt and black pepper

Method:

1. In a large bowl, mix the kale, strawberries and walnuts.
2. Pour the vinegar and olive oil over the salad.

3. Season with salt and black pepper.

Recipe 8: Cinnamon Roll Fat Bombs

Ingredients:

1 teaspoon cinnamon

1 tablespoon coconut oil

2 tablespoons almond butter

½ cup coconut cream

Method:

1. Mix the cinnamon and the coconut cream.
2. Line a suitable baking pan with parchment paper and spread the cinnamon and coconut cream mixture.
3. Mix ½ a teaspoon of cinnamon with coconut oil and almond butter and spread over the first layer in the baking pan.
4. Freeze for about 10 minutes then cut into the desired squares or circular pieces.

Recipe 9: Homemade Chicken Strips

Ingredients:

1 pound of boneless chicken breasts trimmed to finger-like pieces

2 eggs

1 tablespoon of salt

1 teaspoon of freshly ground pepper

1 teaspoon of paprika

1 teaspoon of garlic

2 tablespoons of coconut oil

Hot sauce

Method:

1. Preheat the oven to 300°C and line the baking sheet with aluminum foil.
2. Wash the chicken fingers thoroughly and pat dry using some kitchen towels.
3. In a small bowl, combine the pork rinds, salt, pepper, paprika and garlic. Pour the mixture into a sealable bag.
4. In a larger bowl, beat the eggs and dip each fish finger into the egg wash to coat.
5. Add the chicken breasts that are coated with the egg into the sealable bag with the spice mixture.
6. Seal the bag to allow the mixture to coat the chicken.
7. Place the chicken strips on the baking sheet and place them in the oven. Allow to bake for about 10 – 15 minutes.
8. Flip the chicken over and allow it to cook for another 10 – 15 minutes until golden brown in color. Remove the chicken from the oven and allow it to cool for 5 minutes before serving.
9. Serve with some hot sauce on the side.

Recipe 10: Chicken Wings

Ingredients:

2 pounds chicken wings

1 tablespoon of salt

1 teaspoon of paprika

1 teaspoon of freshly ground black pepper

1 tablespoon of baking powder

1 teaspoon of garlic

2 tablespoons of coconut oil

2 tablespoons of hot sauce

Method:

1. Wash the chicken wings and pat dry.
2. In a small bowl, combine the salt, pepper, baking powder, paprika, and garlic.
3. Place the wings in a sealable plastic bag and add the spice mixture.
4. Seal and shake the bag to coat the wings.
5. Preheat a skillet over medium heat and melt the coconut oil in the warm pan.
6. Place the wings in the skillet and cover.
7. Cook for 10 to 12 minutes.
8. Flip the wings and cook for another 10 to 12 minutes, until golden brown.
9. Remove the wings from the heat and let cool for 5 minutes.
10. Coat the wings with hot sauce, if desired.

Recipe 11: Chicken Stuffed Bell-peppers

Ingredients:

1 tablespoon of butter

1 clove garlic, minced

1 small onion, diced

1 teaspoon of paprika

1 teaspoon of salt

½ teaspoon of freshly ground black pepper

1 teaspoon of chili powder

1 cup grape tomatoes, halved

1-pound ground chicken

3 beaten eggs

4 large bell peppers, halved

Instructions:

1. Preheat the oven to 350°F. Line a baking sheet with parchment paper.
2. Melt the butter in a skillet over medium heat. Add the garlic, onion, salt, pepper, paprika, and chili powder, then sauté for 5 to 7 minutes.
3. Add the tomatoes and sauté for another 5 to 7 minutes.
4. Add the ground chicken and cook until golden brown, about 15 minutes, stirring occasionally.
5. Transfer the cooked meat mixture to a medium-sized bowl and slowly mix in the eggs.
6. Lay each bell pepper half cut side up on the prepared baking sheet.
7. Pour the meat and egg mixture into the bell peppers.
8. Place the stuffed peppers in the oven and bake for 60 minutes, until the peppers soften slightly.

Recipe 12: Simple Homemade bacon

Ingredients:

2 pounds pork belly

⅔ cup salt

2 tablespoons of freshly ground black pepper

Any dried herbs and spices

Method:

1. Remove the skin from the pork belly with a very sharp knife. As you remove it, try to keep the skin intact.
2. Rinse the pork belly and pat dry with a kitchen towel.
3. In a small bowl, mix together the salt, pepper, and any dried herbs and spices.
4. Rub the mixture on both sides of the pork belly.
5. Place the pork belly inside a sealed airtight container and store in the refrigerator for 5 to 7 days. The flavor becomes stronger the longer you cure it.
6. Flip the pork belly over every day. (Make sure you wash your hands thoroughly before touching the pork belly.)
7. After 5 to 7 days, remove the pork belly from the refrigerator and rinse off the salt, pepper, and any other herbs and spices. Pat dry.
8. Preheat the oven to 200°F (90°C).
9. Place a roasting rack in a roasting pan. Place the pork belly fat side up on the rack.
10. Bake until the meat reaches an internal temperature of 150°F. This usually takes about an hour and a half to two hours.
11. Remove the pork belly from the oven and let it cool for 30 minutes.
12. Wrap the meat in parchment paper and store in the refrigerator overnight or for 12 hours.

Recipe 13: Grass-Fed Burgers

Ingredients:

½ teaspoon of garlic powder

½ teaspoon of cumin powder

½ pound of ground grass-fed beef liver

½ pound of ground grass-fed beef

Sea salt and pepper to taste

Desired cooking oil

Method:

1. Mix together all ingredients in a bowl and form patties of your desired size.
2. Heat cooking oil over a skillet on medium-high heat.
3. Cook burgers in skillet until desired.
4. Store in a container in the fridge and use within 4 days.

Your Quick Start Action Step:

Once you begin your intermittent fasting diet, you should always schedule time to plan your meals. This, of course, involves creating time to visit the local market to stock up your kitchen cabinets and refrigerator.

This section provides you with guidance on some of the foods that you could include in your meal plan, and those that are strictly forbidden. Hence, this will give you some guidance to help you in meal planning. As a disclaimer, you must note that the foods are not limited to those listed in this section.

Once you begin your intermittent fasting diet, you could choose a recipe from the above list of recipes. Recipes 1 – 3 are mainly prepared when you want to break your fast. The rest of the recipes can be prepared for other times of the day.

The recipes for the intermittent fasting diet are widely available across the internet and print media. As such, do not feel limited to the ones that we have listed in this section. You can always try out different recipes and stick to specific ones, depending on the recipes that you like best.

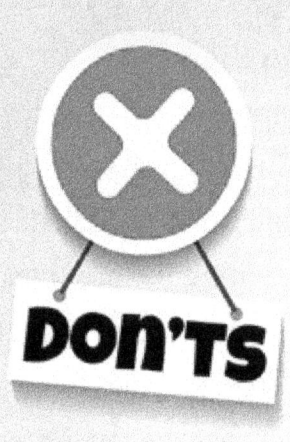

Chapter 10: Mistakes to Avoid and Who Should Not Fast

10.1 Brief Introduction

Many people find intermittent fasting to be an extreme measure and opt for other methods to shed off some of the extra pounds that they want to lose. However, the people who have tried this method can attest to its success in weight loss, and some of the additional benefits that come with it. The method is especially preferred because it ensures that you do not gain the pounds that you have successfully shed off, keeping you healthy lean and fit.

The proponents of this method do however agree that it is difficult, and it is not meant for everyone. This method of weight loss calls for a lot of personal discipline, commitment, and resilience. Throughout the whole process, your willpower will be tested countless times in ways that you cannot imagine or believe to have been possible.

Many people who get on the intermittent fasting diet attest to the fact that getting over the hunger pangs and the food cravings will take a lot of personal discipline and motivation. Most of the time, people are advised to ignore the discomfort that comes with the hunger and instead focus on the goal that they intend to achieve.

However, the hardest part about the whole process is getting over the habit of having three meals each day. Habits are very dangerous because they become ingrained in us and form part of our personality. As such, changing the habit of having three meals a day becomes very difficult.

In addition, the feeling of hunger is controlled by the hormone known as ghrelin. The natural circadian rhythm, which controls the release of the ghrelin hormone, does not follow the eat/fast routine of the intermittent fasting diet. As such, you may find that the moments in which the quantity of the ghrelin hormone is high coincide with your fasting window.

However, here's a piece of encouragement: the beginning is the hardest part, it gets better! All you will need to do is to maintain a positive mindset and surround yourself with positive people, preferably those who share the same goals as you. In no time at all, you will find yourself able to fast for longer hours of time without experiencing any feelings of hunger or cravings.

10.2 A List of People Who Should Not Fast

Based on the extreme nature of the intermittent fasting diet, it is not suitable for everyone. If you have read this book and are attracted to the potential benefits that this diet has in relation to your health and general wellbeing, then you are advised to seek the advice of a medical practitioner or nutritionist.

When you begin the fasting process, you will need to carefully monitor your body for any signs of weakness, dizziness, light-headedness, moodiness, or even constipation. If you observe these symptoms, you are advised to stop the fasting diet and consult the experts on the way forward. The suffering and discomfort that you will experience is simply not worth it.

Pregnant and lactating women are strongly advised against intermittent fasting. This is because they have additional energy needs for the growing fetus and, in the case of lactating women, for the growing baby who depends on breast milk for nourishment. Such women are advised to try out the diet once they have given birth and have breastfed for at least 6 months.

People who have a history of eating disorders are also strongly advised against trying out the intermittent fasting diet. This is because such people already have a history of abnormal and disturbed eating habits, which include anorexia and bulimia nervosa. Fasting may create additional problems for you which may make your situation worse than it already was.

If you are chronically stressed, then it probably is not a good idea for you to create additional stress for your body. The elevated heart rate, high blood pressure, and high levels of stress hormones from chronic stress are already taking a toll on your body. Fasting periods are only going to make your body more stressed and you may not achieve your intended goals.

People who have both type 1 and type 2 diabetes are generally advised against intermittent fasting. In some situations, fasting has led to an increase in blood pressure, and the cholesterol levels in the body, while in other situations, it has reduced the insulin levels and the blood pressure levels. As such, if you are interested in intermittent fasting, you are advised to seek the advice of your doctor.

Anyone who does not get the recommended eight hours of sleep is highly advised to avoid fasting. Inadequate sleep already stresses the body and affects your health. Fasting is likely to make your body deteriorate further. As such, you are more likely to experience feelings of weakness and lightheadedness.

If your lifestyle does not fit into the intermittent fasting process, you should avoid forcing yourself to adopt it. This is because essentially, it is the intermittent diet that is supposed to fit into your life and not the other way around.

Lastly, you should not get on the intermittent fasting diet if you are not interested and most of all passionate about it. Being an extremely demanding process, you will only set yourself up for failure and misery.

10.3 Mistakes to Avoid When Fasting

If you are passionate about intermittent fasting as a tool to lose weight and you convince yourself to give it a try, then there are many pitfalls that you will need to avoid if you are going to be successful. Below are some of the most common mistakes when it comes to intermittent fasting:

1. Inasmuch as intermittent fasting is hard, many people come in with this preconceived notion and end up throwing in the towel too soon. The truth of the matter is that the beginning is the hardest part, it gets better! All you will need to do is to maintain a positive mindset and surround yourself with positive people, preferably those who share the same goals as you. In no time at all, you will find yourself able to fast for longer hours of time without experiencing any feelings of hunger or cravings.

2. On the flip side of the coin, many other people approach the diet with a can-do mentality and end up jumping in way too fast. The problem with this is that such people will set very unrealistic goals, which will end up discouraging them altogether. As such, beginners are advised to start with small but attainable goals which will keep them motivated.

3. Beginners who are just trying out the intermittent fasting process will often put their lives on hold and exclusively focus on fasting to lose weight. This is a mistake, as you will notice the hunger that you are feeling and get tempted to grab a meal during your fasting period. Essentially, you should keep yourself busy to take your mind off your stomach until it is time to break your fast.

4. While there are many ways in which you could go about the intermittent fasting diet, many people often lack guidance, and end up choosing a wrong plan which will only serve to stress you out and make you miserable. As I have repeated several times, the intermittent diet is supposed to fit into your lifestyle and not the other way around. This is the only way in which the habit will stick.

5. Since you will not get many opportunities to eat, both the quantity and quality of the food that you eat will be very important in determining

the success of your fast. Due to the extreme nature of the fast, people often tend to feed on anything they come across without considering its nutritional content, a habit that could easily result in weight gain. As a general rule of thumb, your food should contain healthy portions of all the macronutrients. Starches and simple sugars should however be minimized in order to keep the body in a state of ketosis.

6. People often forget to remain hydrated, most especially during the fasting window. People forget that it is acceptable to have beverages such as mineral water, unsweetened teas, and coffees while fasting. As a matter of fact, these drinks are extremely important as they help to keep hunger at bay and reduce the cravings.

7. When the time to break the fast comes, many people binge eat and feast to make up for the hunger that they experienced during the fasting window. This is a mistake because binge eating will cause your blood sugar levels to sharply increase. Once you resume your fast, the blood sugar levels will also sharply decrease. The fluctuations in the blood sugar levels will lead to moodiness, weakness, and dizziness, which will make it harder to stick to the diet. It is recommended that you should break your fast on a meal that contains 300 – 400 calories.

8. Some people fail to eat enough during the feeding window. Due to lack of knowledge and the fear that they will undo the benefits that they have gained from the fast, many people will eat less than the required amounts. As such, the body will kick into starvation mode by cannibalizing your muscle mass and slowing down your metabolism. This will make it even more difficult to lose weight.

9. Some people may decide to take the whole intermittent fasting process too far, making it difficult to stick to it. Essentially, methods such as the 16/8 method, eat-stop-eat method, and 5:2 method are meant for beginners as you will only need to fast for relatively shorter periods of time. People who decide to begin with the 4:3 method or the 3:3 method often take it too far and end up giving up.

10. Due to all the rage that is associated with intermittent fasting, many

people often try out the method hoping to lose weight quickly and gain the associated benefits. However, some people end up forcing the process to work so much so that they forget that weight loss is a three-part process that involves a positive mindset and physical activity, in addition to the diet. Hence, people forget that there are many other ways of losing weight that do not necessarily involve fasting.

11. The constant, and to some extent, obsessive fear of the feeling of hunger is yet another mistake that people make. People often fear that the body will waste away, and they will die even before the fasting window comes to an end. As such, they respond to the slightest form of hunger by breaking the fast and eventually do not gain anything from the fasting process. Instead, people should avoid any feelings of hunger and rely on the body to produce ketones as an alternative source of fuel.

Your Quick Start Action Step:

Essentially, anyone can take part in intermittent fasting, apart from the people that have been mentioned in the list above. If you are lucky enough to be able to take part in the diet, I would advise you learn from the mistakes of others, as it is only a fool who insists on making their own mistakes.

You are therefore advised to take into consideration some of the common mistakes that have been highlighted and avoid these pitfalls.

Chapter 11: When You Are Not Seeing Results

11.1 Expect That Not All the Results Will Happen

Intermittent fasting is widely famed for all the benefits that it is believed to offer the human body. Some of these benefits include: weight loss, reduced inflammation, improved mental functionality, decreased blood sugar levels, increased insulin sensitivity, and the retarded growth of tumors.

However, human bodies are inherently different, and each body reacts differently to the intermittent fasting process. Some people who fast for extended durations of time may reap all these benefits, some people may reap only a few of these benefits, and others will reap none at all.

If you end up reaping all the benefits, then congratulations to you! If you only reap some of the benefits or even none at all, take courage. Take this as an opportunity to go back to the drawing board to analyze some of the mistakes that you may have made that could have prevented you from reaping these benefits. In addition, make sure to consult a medical practitioner or nutritionist to advise you on the way forward.

One of the main reasons why the fasting process may have failed is that you did not focus on the foods that you were consuming. It could be that you focused on consuming all the wrong foods and did not pay attention to the foods that are required for the intermittent fasting process. Consuming foods that are rich in starches and simple sugars might have caused you to gain weight as opposed to losing it.

Alternatively, it could be that you either consumed too much food or too little food whenever you broke your fast. Consuming little food might have caused your body's metabolism to slow down resulting in an inability to break down fats. Binge eating, otherwise known as feasting, may have increased the calories that you consumed, leading to weight gain as opposed to loss.

Alternatively, you could have chosen a method that could not work for your lifestyle, and that made it extremely difficult for you to follow through with it. You might also have been too aggressive in your approach towards intermittent fasting which may have made it impossible for you to achieve your goals.

In addition, you may find that you were not motivated or enthusiastic about intermittent fasting which greatly affected your morale, making it impossible to achieve some of the goals that you were hoping to. This could have occurred if you were simply following the crowd.

On the other hand, you may have done everything perfectly but still failed to achieve the results that you were hoping for. If this is the case, intermittent fasting is probably not suitable for you. You may want to consider other methods of weight loss which are equally as effective and beneficial to your health and general wellbeing.

You must also be aware that some of these results may take longer to manifest in your body compared to other people. This is because we are all genetically different and some of our biological processes may differ greatly from one person to the next. This should not be a cause for alarm but, instead, a call for you to exercise patience and constancy in the pursuit of your goal.

11.2 Importance of Being Aware of This

Being aware that some of the results may take time to manifest is very important, as it will keep you optimistic and enthusiastic about the intermittent fasting process. It will keep you from giving up and probably motivate you to push your boundaries even further to test your limits.

In addition, knowledge that it is not all the results that will manifest on everyone is important as it will keep you from bad-mouthing the entire fasting process and will allow other people to explore the method without feeling discouraged by your results. In some situations, being aware of this will place you in a better position to advise and motivate others, especially beginners.

11.3 What to Do When the Results Do Not Happen

1. The first thing that you should do if you do not get the results that you intended is to get back to the drawing board and carefully analyze all the steps that you took, being careful to identify any mistakes that you could have made in the process. To make the examination thorough, you could seek the help of a friend to help you to go through the entire process.

2. Once this is done, you should list down all the mistakes that you made and conduct extensive and in-depth research on the correct way to go about these processes. As always, knowledge is power, and the process of learning never stops!

3. You could also seek the advice of your doctor, a medical practitioner, or a nutritionist to provide you with useful insights as to why the process did not work. It could be that you are suffering from a pre-existent condition which made it difficult to follow through with the fasting process, which prevented some of results from happening.

4. If you still believe in intermittent fasting as the key to weight loss, you could join a group of people who are fasting for the same purpose. This will ensure that you have people that you can compare notes with, and who can motivate you to hit your goals whenever you get side-tracked. Alternatively, you could simply request a family member or a friend to become your accountability partner.

5. When the results do not happen because of a poor diet, you could work on improving your fasting diet. First, you could go shopping at your local grocery store or supermarket to source all the ingredients that you will need to prepare healthy and nutritious meals. The foods should have healthy portions of all the major nutrients. Second, take time off your busy schedule to plan for the meals that you will have during each feeding window. Proper meal planning will ensure that you neither under-feed, nor over-feed whenever you break your fast.

6. If you failed to achieve your results due to low commitment and motivation, find a way to keep yourself constantly motivated to achieve your goals. This could be through maintaining a spreadsheet that will track all your progress.

7. If you fail to achieve one of your small goals, find a way to pick yourself up and get back on the horse. You must always remember to be kind to yourself. Whenever you achieve, and possibly even surpass your goals, always find a way to pat yourself on the back, either by giving yourself a gift or rewarding yourself with a cheat day to enjoy some of your favorite meals.

8. You could also focus on setting goals that are less ambitious and more realistic. For starters, you should select a fasting method that caters for shorter fasting windows and longer feeding windows. This is because adjusting from your normal life to the fasting diet will ordinarily require a huge paradigm shift, and extreme discipline. This will probably make it more possible to achieve your goals.

9. Nonetheless, it is important to never force the process on yourself or on your life. If it does not flow naturally, or fit into your lifestyle, then it is probably time that you admitted this to yourself and found alternative ways to lose the weight, and to gain the additional benefits that come with intermittent fasting. The good news is that there are plenty of dietary plans which are available out there, and still as effective. Physical activity and exercises are also recommended. For some of the added benefits, you could use various supplements which will boost your health in the process.

Your Quick Start Action Step:

As such, whenever you fail to achieve the results you had hoped for, you will need to remember that it is not the end of the world, and that there are many more ways that you could use to achieve your goals.

Refer to the above steps which will guide you on some of the areas that you can improve on, and if not, other recommended ways of shedding off the extra pounds, and enjoying the results of the fasting diet without necessarily being on one.

Bearing this in mind, you must pick yourself up, dust yourself off, put on a brave face, and go forth to correct some of the mistakes that you might have made. Again, you must never forget that fasting is indeed a lifestyle and not merely a one-time thing. This will help you to realize that most of the results will not be achieved in the blink of an eye, nor will they be achieved in a couple of weeks, or months. You will need to persistently and diligently put in the effort, while setting your sights on the bigger goal that you aim to achieve.

You will also need to remember that the intermittent fasting diet will require your time in meal planning and meal preparation. Hence, always make sure to schedule time in the course of your busy day to do these activities which are likely to make all the difference.

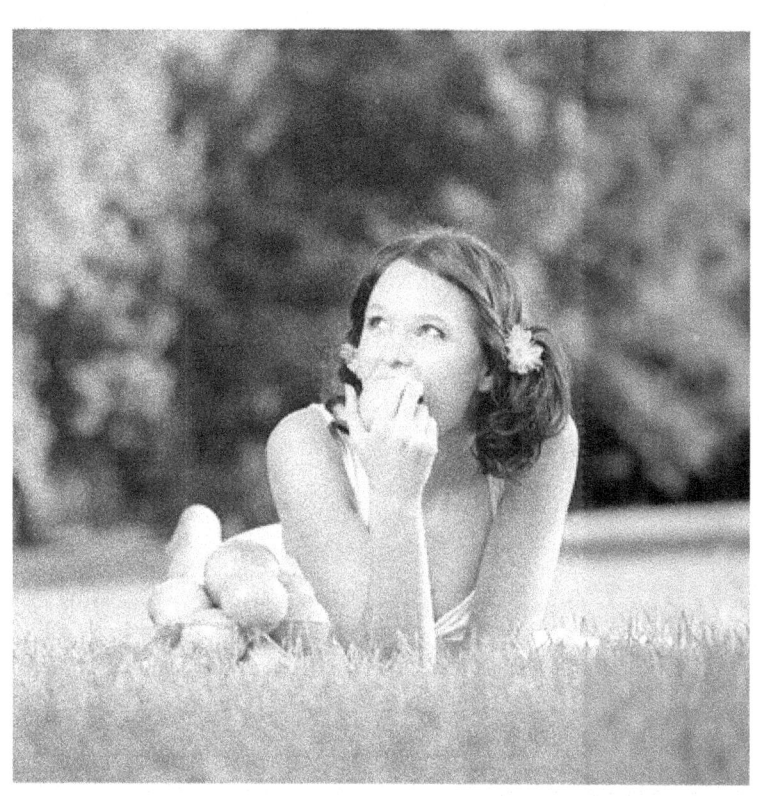

Chapter 12: Living the Healthy, Guilt-Free Lifestyle

12.1 Intermittent Fasting as a Lifestyle

By now, you must have realized that despite the hype and the craze that is associated with the intermittent fasting diet, one important fact that many people fail to consider is that fasting is not merely a dietary plan, or a one-hit-wonder. It is a lifestyle, a way of life.

Intermittent fasting uses a holistic way in approaching the problem of weight loss. It is a three-part process that encompasses your mindset, the fitness and exercise levels, and most of all, your dietary plan, which is where the intermittent fasting diet comes in.

As such, the benefits of this diet are not merely weight loss, but include increasing insulin sensitivity, reducing blood sugar levels, reducing inflammations in the body, longevity and slow aging, increased metabolism, and the retarded growth of cancer cells.

Despite being one of the fastest and most effective methods of losing weight, optimal results will only be expected when you combine the diet with healthy nutrition and a healthy lifestyle.

The foods that you consume should be rich in important minerals, vitamins, and other nutrients which are important in ensuring proper bodily functions. Junk foods, foods that are rich in starch and simple sugars, carbonated drinks, white refined foods, and fatty cuts of meat are generally considered unhealthy and should not be consumed while on the intermittent fasting diet.

Physical exercise and workouts are also highly recommended, despite the low energy levels that are experienced while fasting. These exercises are mainly recommended for individuals who have been on the diet for a while and are comfortable in fasting. The exercise should not be intensive but should stretch the bodily organs and make sure that the muscles are well toned. This will prevent saggy skin after the weight loss.

The mindset is also an important aspect of the intermittent fasting process. In general, one's mindset should be very positive and optimistic when going into this diet. A few weeks or months into the diet, you will learn the important skills of resilience and personal discipline, which will serve to strengthen your willpower and contribute to making you a better person.

12.2 Why Intermittent Fasting is Worth it in the End

While it is unanimously agreed upon that intermittent fasting is a daunting and difficult task, proponents of the method still believe that it is one of the most effective weight loss programs, as it often improves on different aspects of your general lifestyle and wellbeing. Once you achieve some of these goals or results, the trouble that you went through while fasting becomes insignificant.

Below are some of the reasons why intermittent fasting is worth it:

Unlike most other dietary plans and fasting methods, none guarantees people that they will not regain the weight that they have lost. These methods only cater for the weight loss part and leave the maintenance of the new weight to you. Seeing as many people fail to maintain their new weight on their own, the intermittent fasting diet tops the list.

Intermittent fasting is unique as it results in an extended lifespan. Intermittent fasting diets are believed to alter the mitochondrial networks inside the energy producing cells, increasing lifespan, and promoting good health.

The intermittent fasting diet has also been proven to have benefits for patients suffering from type 2 diabetes. As a result of the decreased insulin levels in the bloodstream, the cells become more sensitive to any insulin released into the bloodstream. As such, it does not accumulate within the blood. This then leads to an improvement in insulin sensitivity.

The growth of carcinogenic tumors is also retarded. Periodic fasting leads to a decrease in the growth of cancerous tumors and increased sensitivity to chemotherapy. When cancerous cells are exposed to environments that contain lower glucose levels, proliferation and cell death quickly follow, a process known as cell starvation.

Through intermittent fasting, we have a significant decrease in inflammation in the body. Inflammation is a common symptom of all chronic diseases that we face today. It is known to occur whenever the body is trying to heal itself. However, whenever inflammation occurs for too long, it is associated with some negative effects.

Improved brain functionality and cognitive functions also comes up when the body uses ketones as sources of energy, as opposed to the conventional glucose.

12.3 Steps on How to Maintain a Healthy Lifestyle

1. One should focus on eating healthy meals and drinking calorie-free drinks such as water, unsweetened teas, and coffee. Feeding on unhealthy meals that consist of soft drinks, energy drinks, meals that are rich in simple starches, saturated fats and oils, and white foods is extremely detrimental to your body.
2. Boost your intake of fruits and vegetables. Fruits and vegetables are an important constituent of a healthy diet. They are rich in nutrients, minerals and phytonutrients, which boost the individual's immunity and help to fight disease-causing organisms.
3. Consume foods that are rich in fibers. Fibers often absorb water when in the gut. This causes them to become soft and bulky. This reduces constipation by making the bowel movements easier.
4. Cut down on processed foods. These foods are often stripped of important nutrients and replaced with synthetic nutrients. Some of them even contain preservatives, which may be harmful to your health. Opt for organic foods as opposed to processed foods.
5. Choose white meats over red meats. Red meats have been linked to increased risk of colon cancer, and increased cholesterol levels. White

meats on the other hand are very nutritious. Fish for example is rich in omega-3 oils and vitamin D.

6. Keep your body physically fit and well-toned by visiting the gym, taking long walks, participating in yoga, or carrying out simple exercises from the comfort of your own home. Depending on your age, medical factors, ethnicity, and other factors, you could choose between low, moderate, and high-intensity exercises.

7. Maintain a healthy weight, and by extension, a healthy Body Mass Index (BMI). A healthy Body Mass Index is found anywhere between 18.5 and 24.9.

8. Avoid smoking and restrict your alcohol intake as much as possible. Smoking is generally unhealthy, as it leads to many other diseases and complications. As such, it should be avoided at all costs.

9. Avoid eating very heavy meals at a go. Instead, focus on consuming light meals at frequent intervals. This will keep your blood sugar levels in check and prevent the feelings of drowsiness and moodiness that often come with unstable levels of blood sugar.

10. Replace saturated fats with unsaturated fats. Saturated fats have the potential of increasing your cholesterol levels. This is harmful to your health and could result in cardiovascular disease and other heart diseases.

11. Keep your body hydrated by consuming plenty of mineral water, freshly squeezed juices, and calorie-free drinks. Essentially, you should drink at least eight glasses of water each day. This will keep your skin supple and your body organs functional.

12. Reduce your intake of salts and sugar. Salt has the potential of increasing your blood pressure, as well as the risk of cardiovascular diseases, and other heart diseases. When shopping, try to identify foods that are low in sodium. In addition, avoid adding salt at the dinner table. Although sugar is sweet and attractive, it should only be enjoyed in moderation as it could lead to high blood pressure.

13. Meet your daily sleep requirements. Sleep is an important factor that is often overlooked. Sleep gives your body rest by helping your muscles to recover. In addition, it keeps you looking younger and prevents you from aging! You should always aim for 6 – 7 hours of sleep every night.
14. Take time off your busy schedule to meditate. This will quieten down your body and soul and allow them to be one. This is especially important for concentration.

Your Quick Start Action Step:

Living a healthy lifestyle is a process that not only involves your dietary intake, but also your physical activity levels and your ability to stick to the process.

To live a healthy lifestyle, you should consider following the above-mentioned steps. The most important part about following these steps is having a can-do-mentality and remaining committed throughout the process. This could be achieved by surrounding yourself with like-minded people who will push you towards a healthy lifestyle.

In as much as the list above provides a conclusive list of some of the steps that you could take to live a healthy lifestyle, you must realize that it is not exclusive and there are many other steps that you could take to maintain a healthy lifestyle.

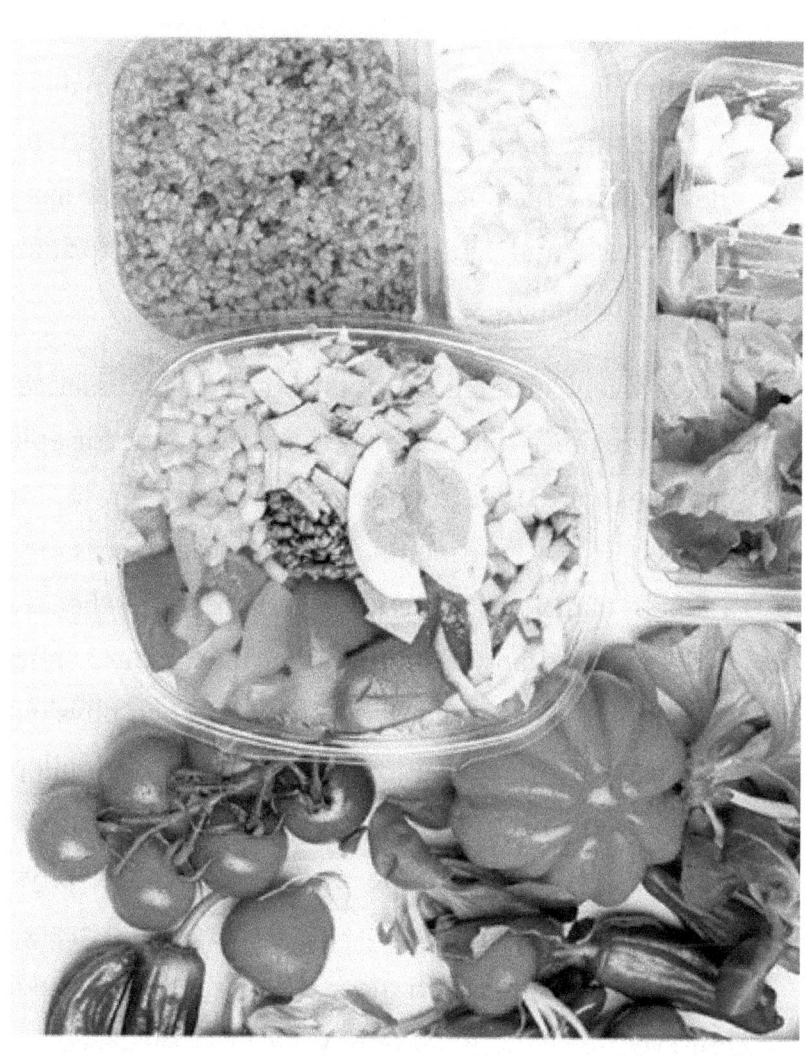

Bonus Chapter: Benefits with Ketogenic Diet

12.1 Background Information on the Ketogenic Diet

You've probably heard of the phrase 'keto diet' used amongst fitness experts and other individuals looking to hit their fitness goals. The ketogenic diet, often shortened to the keto diet, has become one of the most popular ways to shed off a few extra kilos. Despite its recent hype, the diet has been used by medical experts for more than one hundred years. It was initially popularized in the early 1920s and 1930s as a dietary therapy for epileptic patients. Today, the diet has proven benefits for weight loss, and the general health and performance of epileptic and diabetic patients.

The ketogenic diet has its roots in the ancient practice of fasting, and other dietary regimes that were used as treatment for epilepsy. These ancient practices were used from as early as 500 B.C., in the days of the ancient Greeks. These treatments included the excess or limitation of some animal, plant, or mineral substances. In the early 1920s, modern physicians began to mimic the biochemical effects of fasting and starvation to treat epilepsy. A pair of French physicians, were the first to record the use of starvation as a treatment for epilepsy. The pair treated 20 children and adults and reported that the seizures were less during the treatment period. For the next two decades, physicians and medical doctors conducted widespread research and tests on this method of treatment, during which the method was widely used. The use of the diet however declined in the late 1930s after the discovery of anti-convulsant drugs.

In the 1970s, a very low carbohydrate diet for weight loss was popularized by Dr. Atkins in his paper. The diet began with a two-week ketogenic phase that allowed for zero intake of carbohydrates. This was followed by a gradual addition of carbohydrates that ensured that the body kept burning its fat as fuel. Hence, individuals would continue to lose without hunger. In the long-term, individuals were to engage in meals containing 60% fats, 30% protein, and 10% carbohydrates. However, the followers of Atkin's diet were at a risk of having cancer, constipation, and malnutrition, amongst other health risks. Today, many years later, many fad diets still incorporate the same approach to weight loss.

That said, what then is a ketogenic diet? The ketogenic diet is a high-fat, low-carb, and moderate-protein meal plan. It entails eating foods that are rich in fats and reducing the intake of carbohydrates. It typically includes foods such as: meat, eggs, cheese, milk, processed meat, nuts, butter, oils, and seeds.

In the presence of carbohydrates, the body normally converts carbohydrates into glucose, which is then transported throughout the body to provide energy to perform different bodily functions. However, in the absence of carbohydrates, the liver breaks down fats into fatty acids and ketone bodies. The ketone bodies are then passed into the bloodstream, replacing glucose as a source of energy. As such, the body burns fats rather than carbohydrates to produce energy, a state known as ketosis. Generally, with a carbohydrate intake of less than 20 to 50 grams per day, the body takes about two to four days to shift from using circulating glucose to breaking down stored fats for energy.

While on a ketogenic diet, the body switches from glucose to ketones as the primary source of fuel supply. The body then increases the burning of fat, leading to a significant decrease in insulin levels in the bloodstream. This then becomes important to individuals who are trying to lose weight, for it makes it easier for the body to access and burn off fat reserves without the feeling of hunger or a decrease in the supply of energy, as is common with people who are fasting. However, it is argued that a ketogenic diet is more of a short-term diet that a long-term lifestyle. This is because of the social restrictions that the diet imposes on an individual.

Scientific research also indicates that weight loss results after being on a ketogenic diet for 12 months are the same as those of individuals on a healthy diet.

In addition to people who are trying to lose weight, the ketogenic diet is also important to people with type 2 diabetes. Ketogenic diets assist the body in controlling blood sugar levels by reducing the amount of glucose in the bloodstream. This is known as glycemic control. As a result, the diet reduces the amount of insulin medication that a patient is required to take. However, keeping in mind that ketogenic diets include a high intake of fats, if the fats are saturated or of poor quality, then this may put a patient at a risk for cardiovascular diseases. A fat saturated diet leads to an increase in harmful cholesterol, placing one at a risk of heart problems. As such, people with type 2 diabetes are required to consult with their doctors before getting on a ketogenic diet.

There is also solid evidence dating back to more than one hundred years that seems to point out that, indeed, a ketogenic diet does reduce epileptic seizures especially in children. Because of these neuroprotective effects, physicians and medical doctors have been investigating any possible benefits for other brain disorders such as autism, Alzheimer's, and even Parkinson's disease. Hence, the ketogenic diet has proven to be important to people suffering from epilepsy.

The ketogenic diet, as we have seen, is a very important alternative in treating diabetes and epilepsy as well as in weight loss. However, the diet could become unhealthy if individuals partake in too much red meat, fatty foods, processed foods, and salty foods. These foods have the potential to complicate the situation further by introducing other complications such as heart problems. However, a balanced and unprocessed ketogenic diet that is rich in lean meats, fish, nuts, olive oils, seeds, whole grains, fruits, and vegetables is more likely to lead to a long and happy life.

The ketogenic diet is often used interchangeably with the intermittent fasting diet. This is because the condition of being overweight, and by extension, obesity, is mainly caused by the insulin hormone in the bloodstream. Being a fat storage hormone, whenever you consume more calories than your body needs, the insulin levels will rise and will stimulate the body to store the excess glucose as fat reserves within the body, leading to weight gain.

Hence, the ketogenic diet and the intermittent fasting diet are mainly based on the principle of reducing the insulin levels in the bloodstream to prevent the accumulation of fat deposits. Both diets also boost the ketone levels in the bloodstream and make the body burn more fats. When used simultaneously, these two methods are guaranteed to boost your weight loss and to improve your health and general wellbeing.

While it is true that you can use each of these methods independently, you will realize that it is more practical to use them simultaneously rather than independently. This is because intermittent fasting while on a ketogenic diet gives a significant boost to your weight loss journey, and vice versa is consequently true.

12.2 The Link between Intermittent Fasting and the Keto Diet

Having noted that intermittent fasting and the ketogenic diet affect the body in the same way, we will need to explore the link between these two methods of weight loss to understand just why it is that they work together so well.

Recall that the ketogenic diet is a high-fat, low-carb, and moderate-protein meal plan that results in a state of ketosis. By consuming fewer carbohydrates, there is less glucose, and by extension, less insulin in the bloodstream. The body then burns down its fat reserves to release energy in the form of ketones. Increased fat loss then results in weight loss.

Hence, keto dieters will have low blood sugar and low insulin levels. They will also be fully into the fat-burning mode, ketosis. The elevated ketones in the bloodstream and the satiating effects of the ketogenic diet will result in a reduced appetite, less hunger pangs, and cravings. These effects will especially be beneficial to people who are practicing intermittent fasting.

The ketogenic diet is believed to result in hunger suppression, which is important to people practicing intermittent fasting. The elevated ketones in the body suppress the production of the ghrelin hormone. The ghrelin hormone is based on the natural circadian rhythm and is responsible for hunger. Low levels of ghrelin reduce the feeling of hunger, even when you do not have any food in your system. As such, you can go for longer without eating anything and fasting becomes easier.

As mentioned earlier, the ketogenic diet is rich in fats and oils. Fats and oils do not spike your blood sugar levels. Instead, they stabilize the sugar levels. As such, pairing a ketogenic diet with intermittent fasting will result in stable and low blood sugar levels. This will eliminate any fatigue, mood swings, and cravings that may be associated with high-carb fasting. As such, combining the two methods could be especially useful to people suffering from type 2 diabetes.

In addition, high-carb diets will cause your blood sugar levels to rise whenever you break your fast, and to drop significantly during your fasting window. Unstable blood sugar levels will negatively impact the intermittent fasting process as they will result in sleepiness, low energy, mood swings, and intense cravings. If this keeps happening, intermittent fasting becomes very difficult. The intense hunger will cause you to binge eat, or to feast whenever you break your fast. Consuming the additional calories will then cause you to gain weight as opposed to losing it.

The low-carb ketogenic diet also results in mental sharpness and acuity. There is plenty of scientific evidence that seems to suggest that ketones improve our cognitive abilities and mental functioning. The western diet, which typically consists of foods that are rich in refined carbohydrates, has been proven to result in the degradation of the nervous system, resulting in reduced memory and cognitive abilities.

In addition, ketones are believed to boost mental abilities since they are a much more efficient source of energy. Fats are more powerful because they contain much more energy for every unit of oxygen that is utilized. Glucose is used up more quickly compared to fats. As such, fat is a more constant source of energy for the brain.

Intermittent fasting is also beneficial to the ketogenic diet. The cycles of the eating and fasting windows ensure that the insulin levels in the bloodstream are low, resulting in higher ketone levels in the bloodstream. Higher ketone levels convert the body into a fat-burning machine resulting in weight loss.

Furthermore, intermittent fasting works through calorie restriction. The methods of intermittent fasting ensure that your daily calorie intake is significantly less than what a normal person on a three-meal-a-day approach is consuming because of the restricted feeding window. Better still, some methods of intermittent fasting ensure that your calorie intake is low whether you are feeding on healthy and nutritious meals, or unhealthy meals. Hence, intermittent fasting allows you to restrict your calorie intake while on the ketogenic diet.

Intermittent fasting also leads to the production of a protein called brain-derived neurotrophic factor (BDNF) within the nerve cells. The protein leads to improved learning, memory, and increases the production of new nerve cells. Animal studies have found that it also makes brain neurons resistant to dysfunction and degeneration.

12.3 How to Maximize the Benefits of Both Intermittent Fasting and the Ketogenic Diet

There are many benefits that you will expect to enjoy when you combine the ketogenic diet with intermittent fasting. They include: reduced hunger and cravings, increased energy levels, reduced moodiness and crankiness, improved mental functionality, increased insulin sensitivity, lower blood sugar, and efficient weight loss.

To enjoy these benefits, you will need to put in place some steps and measures that will ensure that you maximize these benefits. They are listed below:

1. Consult your medical practitioner before you start. This is especially the case if you suffer from any known medical conditions, such as diabetes and high blood pressure, if you are pregnant, or if you are breastfeeding.

2. Set your goals: You will need to analyze your eating habits, current weight, and any health conditions that you may have. Then create a game plan that involves the combination of the ketogenic diet and intermittent fasting, which will lead you to your goal. Inasmuch as losing weight is the ultimate goal, individuals should create smaller milestones to motivate them to move closer to the goal.

3. Surround yourself with positive energy: Avoid keeping the company of people who persistently remind you of your weight. Instead, surround yourself with people who are positive, and encourage you to become your best self. For added motivation, you could join a slimming club, which is a great way to meet new people who share the same goals as you.

4. Make sure your goals are realistic and attainable: Remember that the journey of a thousand miles starts with a single step. It doesn't matter how small you start, just as long as you start. This will provide you with a platform to work towards your ultimate goal.

5. Keep track of all your activities: You could track yourself using a food diary, an exercise log, or a spreadsheet that contains both records. By keeping track of your fitness exercises, eating habits, and even your moods, you become more accountable to yourself, and are motivated to achieve your next goal.

6. The ketogenic diet primarily involves the consumption of meals that contain high amounts of fats and oils, moderate amounts of protein, and low amounts of carbohydrates. Generally, the meals should also minimize the total calories which are being consumed. To maximize

the weight loss process, you must ensure that all ingredients that you select meet the above criteria. This will reduce the glucose levels in the bloodstream, and consequently, the levels of insulin. As such, the body will turn to its fat reserves as a source of fuel. The burning of fats will then result in weight loss.

7. The amount of carbohydrates that you consume should be minimized as much as possible. This is because feeding on high-carb foods while fasting intermittently will cause your blood sugar levels to rise whenever you break your fast, and to drop significantly during your fasting window. Unstable blood sugar levels will negatively impact the intermittent fasting process, as they will result in sleepiness, low energy, mood swings, and intense cravings.

8. Ketosis is a process that allows the body to burn down its fat reserves as a source of energy and fuel. When high-carb foods are broken down, glucose is released into the bloodstream and the body reverts to its natural state of breaking down glucose for energy. As such, you should avoid high-carb foods because they terminate the process of ketosis and could result in weight gain, which goes against your main objective for intermittent fasting.

9. High fats and oils in the ketogenic diet are important to the intermittent fasting process because they provide the muscles and body organs with all the important minerals and nutrients that are required. In addition, fats and oils keep you satiated, reducing the occurrence of hunger pangs and cravings, which greatly impacts an individual's ability to fast for long periods of time. Fats and oils also result in improved mental performance and a reduction in inflammation.

10. While the ketogenic diet allows for foods that contain high fats, moderate proteins, and low carbohydrates, you should always abstain from eating unhealthy fats and proteins. Saturated fats have the potential of increasing your cholesterol levels. This is harmful to your health and could result in cardiovascular disease and other heart

diseases. You should therefore avoid eating the following foods: fatty cuts of beef and pork, foods that have been deep fried, some dairy products such as cream, cheese, and butter.

11. The ketogenic diet should therefore be well balanced and should largely contain unprocessed foods. Some of the foods that are recommended include: lean cuts of beef, pork, lamb and goat meat, fish, nuts, olive oils, seeds, whole grains, fruits, and vegetables. Such a diet is extremely nutritious and is likely to result in the longevity of your life, improved immunity, and reduced constipation.

12. Calorie-free beverages are also very important as they provide you with the desired hydration to keep your body in perfect shape. Coffee is particularly considered to be very important as it increases the metabolism of the body, leading to the increased burning of fat as a source of energy. In addition, coffee is important in reducing hunger pangs and cravings.

13. Identify the days of the week and schedule specific periods in the course of the day or the week in which you will have your meals, or those in which you will fast. The timings can always be changed depending on your schedule and bodily needs.

14. Repeat the process. As mentioned earlier, the ketogenic diet and intermittent fasting are a way of life, and you cannot expect the results to be visible within one day, one week, or even one month. The intended results will come as a result of consistency and dedication in the pursuit of your goal.

15. The first meal of the day, which is meant to break the fast, should be modest in size. Breaking the fast with a very large meal, or through binge eating, will slow down the fat burning process in your body making you tired. As such, the first meal that you consume after breaking your fast should contain 300 – 500 calories.

Your Quick Start Action Step:

Schedule some time to carry out in depth research and to consult a medical practitioner to provide you with all the knowledge that you will need before starting the ketogenic diet and intermittent fasting. This is especially so if you are suffering from any known medical conditions such as diabetes and high blood pressure, if you are pregnant, or breastfeeding. Armed with the necessary knowledge, you could follow the steps highlighted above to schedule your fasting and feeding window, to create a suitable meal plan and to plan any workouts that you plan to engage in. To create a comprehensive and conclusive meal plan, you will need to go out and shop for some of these foods and ingredients to restock your refrigerator and kitchen cabinets.

As you pursue this journey, you will need to realize that it is not for everyone. It will test your will and determination countless times. Hence, you will need to constantly motivate yourself and keep the company of positive people, preferably people who are pursuing the same goal. You could also frequently track your progress by recording it in a spreadsheet. If you do not meet your goals, do not be hard on yourself. You will need to realize that fasting is difficult and find ways to motivate yourself to get back on track.

If you feel weak, dizzy, sluggish, moody, constantly tired, or experience some brain fog, you may need to stop the ketogenic diet and intermittent fasting process and seek the advice of your medical practitioner. You will need to realize that all human beings are fundamentally different and run your own race. After all, life is not a competition.

Conclusion

Thank you again for owning this book!

I hope this book was able to help you to understand how intermittent fasting can be used to lose weight, and to live a healthier lifestyle. In addition, I hope that the bonus chapter was helpful in linking intermittent fasting to the ketogenic diet.

So far, I hope you have come to understand that intermittent fasting is not merely a diet, but a way of life that comes with numerous health benefits for you. It is also my hope that you have come to appreciate the benefits that come with the intermittent fasting diet and have come to terms with the fact that it is not as extreme as people make it sound. In addition to the known benefits, you must be aware that intermittent fasting is a new concept, and that there are many more benefits that are still being explored and studied by nutritionist and medical practitioners.

Inasmuch as intermittent fasting and the ketogenic diet are perfect compliments in the weight loss journey, do not feel pressured to adopt both the methods since they still work perfectly when used independently. It is advisable that you begin with the ketogenic diet, then gradually incorporate the intermittent fasting method once you believe in yourself.

If you have started intermittent fasting and it feels uncomfortable at first, I would advise you to give yourself time to adjust. There is no standard duration of time that it will take you to adjust to fasting, as we are all inherently different and unique. Hence, simply monitor your body and understand some of the signals that it will be communicating to you.

Throughout the whole process, you must bear in mind that intermittent fasting will indeed test your discipline and willpower in ways that you cannot imagine or believe to be possible. However, here's a piece of encouragement; the beginning is the hardest part, it gets better! All you will need to do is to maintain a positive mindset and surround yourself with positive people, preferably those who share the same goals as you. In no time at all, you will find yourself able to fast for longer without experiencing any feelings of hunger or cravings.

To keep yourself motivated, you could maintain a record of your feeding habits and physical activities in a spreadsheet to help you monitor your progress, and to establish any trends that could provide opportunities for growth.

It cannot be stressed enough that intermittent fasting is not for everyone! As such, as soon as you begin the fasting process, you will need to carefully monitor your body for any signs of weakness, dizziness, light-headedness, moodiness, or even constipation. If you observe these symptoms, you are advised to stop the fasting diet and consult the experts moving forward.

Beginners should focus on having shorter fasting windows, and gradually work towards increasing the hours, as they gain more resilience and endurance. If you are unable to complete the fasting window without eating, do not be hard on yourself. Instead, take time to re-strategize to ensure that you do not fall again. To avoid breaking your fast prematurely, you could put in place gifting mechanisms where you will reward yourself for successfully completing the fasting window.

Anyone suffering from a health condition should be careful and consult the advice of a medical practitioner before starting the intermittent fasting diet. This is especially the case for people suffering from diabetes or high blood pressure. Such people should persistently monitor their blood sugar levels and blood pressure at least four times daily.

The next step is to implement everything that you have learned from this book. Feel free to make any amendments and modifications to suit you and your lifestyle. After all, you must always remember that the intermittent fasting diet is meant to fit into your life and not the other way around.

Bearing in mind that knowledge is power, you should never stop reading, researching, or consulting on the intermittent fasting diet. Feel free to get the opinions of other people and frequently compare notes with them to stay motivated and optimistic. As such, now that you have successfully completed this book, start researching on the next book that you will be picking up.

Once you have gotten comfortable with intermittent fasting, you could slowly begin to incorporate a workout or fitness program to keep yourself physically fit. Due to the intensity of the program, you will need to only consider activities that are either light or moderate. To get the most out of your fitness program, you could consult a fitness expert who will create a workout plan for you.

In conclusion, you should always bear in mind that you are a social creature, and like all social creatures, you have social needs and demands. Hence, do not avoid going to celebrations or feasts because you are fasting. Occasionally give yourself a break and join other people to make merry. Later, you could compensate for this by fasting for extended periods of time or restructuring your feeding and fasting windows.

Thank you and good luck!

www.ingramcontent.com/pod-product-compliance
Lightning Source LLC
Chambersburg PA
CBHW080213040426

42333CB00044B/2638